ON THIS BRIGHT DAY

A Year of Reflections for Lasting Food Freedom

Susan Peirce Thompson, Ph.D.

HAY HOUSE, INC.
Carlsbad, California • New York City
London • Sydney • New Delhi

Published in the United States by: Hay House, Inc.: www.hayhouse.com® • *Published in Australia by:* Hay House Australia Pty. Ltd.: www.hayhouse.com.au • *Published in the United Kingdom by:* Hay House UK, Ltd.: www.hayhouse.co.uk • *Published in India by:* Hay House Publishers India: www.hayhouse.co.in

Cover design: Julie Davison • *Interior design:* Bryn Starr Best • *Indexer:* J S Editorial, LLC

Cataloging-in-Publication Data is on file at the Library of Congress

Hardcover ISBN: 978-1-4019-5932-6
E-book ISBN: 978-1-4019-5933-3
Audiobook ISBN: 978-1-4019-5936-4

10 9 8 7 6 5 4 3 2 1
1st edition, October 2023

Printed in the United States of America

SUSTAINABLE FORESTRY INITIATIVE

Certified Chain of Custody
Promoting Sustainable Forestry

www.forests.org
SFI-01268

SFI label applies to the text stock

*For those who muster the courage
to surrender the food and recover.
With love and unity.*

INTRODUCTION

Dear Reader,

Welcome to a year of daily meditations created to support and inspire your Bright Journey. I started Bright Line Eating (BLE) in 2015 after two decades in various 12-step food recovery programs. What I saw in some of those rooms were people who had lost all their excess weight and kept it off for decades. As a brain and cognitive scientist teaching a college course on the psychology of eating, I knew that was an anomaly in the weight-loss annals. But more impressive was that those same people had achieved a level of peace around food that those in the throes of food addiction only dream of.

By studying how highly refined foods affect the brain, I was able to connect the dots and explain why and how the sugar and flour in our modern diet hijack the brain and cause us to eat in ways and amounts we never intended, lead us to break our promises to ourselves, and perpetuate the ever-increasing rates of obesity and diabetes we see worldwide.

I knew that if we could offer people a program that enabled them to permanently eliminate sugar and flour from their diets and also address the behavioral addiction component, people's lives could be saved.

To date that has proved true for tens of thousands of people. But like all recovery journeys, it is not easy. If you are among the 20 percent of the population who measure at the very highest end of the Food Addiction Susceptibility Scale (which you can explore at FoodAddictionQuiz.com), getting sober from sugar and flour requires determination, commitment, perseverance, and, above all, support.

This book is intended to offer a daily dose of encouragement and wisdom, whether you are a Bright Lifer, a member of a 12-step community, or just embarking on your own food journey. Perhaps you are standing in a bookstore right now praying for a solution to the daily agony you face, and this book jumped out at you. Welcome.

This book is written with Bright Line Eating language, but feel free to make it your own if you use different words in your program. For those of you unfamiliar with Bright Line Eating, the early entries in January explain the four Bright Lines and the central tenets of the program. And all our core philosophies, habits, and best practices get their turn in the sun as you move through the year.

If you are picking this up midyear, there is a glossary at the back of the book with definitions of popular terms in the Bright community, like NMF (Not My Food), NMD (Not My Drink), BLTs (Bites, Licks, and Tastes), and Rezoom. Rezooming is something we do when we have broken (or bent) one of our Bright Lines. We marshal tremendous compassion for ourselves, get social support, and seek the lesson. Most of all, we resume eating Bright as quickly as possible, with our next meal or even our next bite, hence Re-*zoom!*

As you begin the journey of your Bright Transformation and begin to get clear on your goal, know that Bright Bodies come in a range of shapes and sizes. Their underlying commonality is that they are free of processed sugar and flour, have shed their unhealthy weight, and carry minds that are at peace with food and focused outward on the world at large. Folks who have had—or are eagerly embarking on—their Bright Transformation tend to think of themselves as Bright Lifers, members of the community whose sense of identity is inextricably linked with this new way of eating and the freedom it brings them. They live at what we call Maintenance, a stage where we eat the exact amount of food required to maintain our goal weight and make us feel energetic and peaceful. This stage lasts a lifetime.

Within these pages, you will also encounter language from the Internal Family Systems (IFS) model of the psyche, which works from the premise that the brain or the self isn't one cohesive monolith. Rather, we have parts, and those parts can sometimes be in conflict. In Bright Line Eating we often find that an inner Rebel part of us might buck against the restrictions, while an inner Isolator part might pull us away from getting the support we need. Those parts of us typically came into being as coping mechanisms in childhood, and they do the best they can with the tools they had. Our job now as adults is to ask those parts to trust us, step aside, and allow us to operate from our Authentic Self, which we can recognize when we feel calm, clear, compassionate, confident, creative, curious, courageous, and connected.

In my own journey, books like the one you hold in your hand have been a companion and a comfort. The heart of this path we walk is surrender. We accept that we are powerless over the substance that has mastered us. We accept that the only sane path forward is eliminating it from our lives for today. We accept the help of those who walk ahead, we stand shoulder to shoulder with those on the journey, and we offer a hand to those arriving behind us.

Day by day we feel a little better. Day by day it gets a little easier. Day by day our world gets Brighter.

A Bright year only happens one day at a time.

I welcome you with my whole heart.

Happy Bright New Year!

Love,
Susan Peirce Thompson, Ph.D.

January

BEGINNINGS

You must do the thing you think you cannot do.
— ELEANOR ROOSEVELT

January 1 is probably the most infamous day on the calendar for chronic dieters. A day when the starting gun is fired and change is on the horizon. A day when we psychologically turn over a new leaf, relegating failure to the past and freeing ourselves up to have hope about what is possible.

But as we all know, the Fresh Start Effect is not enough to keep us on track come February or March, much less last the year. For the long term, we need an effective plan and consistent support. All of which is available to you here. Even if in the past, January 1 was a kickoff to a program that did not lead to long-term weight loss or big life changes, right here and right now you can have an effective fresh start, whether you are well into your Bright Journey, just starting off, or recommitting. And that is exciting.

On this fresh new day, acknowledge the courage it takes to eat Bright, and the excitement, hope, anticipation, or even trepidation you may have. All those feelings are welcome. Be awake to what is, accept it, and use it to move toward what you truly want. This yearlong path will help you heal your relationship with food and finally live your fullest, Brightest life possible. In fellowship.

ON THIS BRIGHT DAY,

I COURAGEOUSLY TAKE A SIGNIFICANT
STEP ON MY BRIGHT TRANSFORMATION.

NO SUGAR

Desperate ills need desperate remedies.
— AGATHA CHRISTIE

Many of us have found that our lifelong relationship with sugar has been one of painful, relentless addiction. We sometimes ate until we were sick, and we rarely felt entirely in control. When we did try to moderate our consumption, it required an exhausting level of mental exertion that always ended in sugar re-establishing its dominance over us. Particularly if we're high on the Food Addiction Susceptibility Scale, we learned a truth the hard way: we cannot eat sugar in moderation.

We must remember what sugar does to our brain. It raises insulin levels, blocking leptin, the hormone that makes us feel full—meaning that eating sugar can actually make us feel *insatiably* hungry.

At the end of the day, the only way to attain true liberation is to eliminate this scourge completely. To allow our brain to heal, and watch our heart and soul follow. Because we don't just carry the burden of excess weight; we carry the burden of an addiction that stands between us and everything we aspire to be.

This Bright Line is the birthplace of all you are trying to achieve—in your body and your mind and your life.

ON THIS BRIGHT DAY,
I WILL TAKE THE ROAD THAT LEADS
TO FREEDOM, NO MATTER WHAT.

January 3
NO FLOUR

A hero is someone who understands the
responsibility that comes with his freedom.
— BOB DYLAN

For those of us who are high on the Food Addiction Susceptibility Scale, we must surrender to a truth: flour works the
same way as sugar in the brain. That is to say, addictively. Refined
foods hit our bloodstream and create the same dopamine spike
and insulin cascade as sugar. For this reason, many of us have not
had success staying off sugar when we were still eating flour—
consuming flour, no matter what kind, can keep that cycle of
cravings alive.

What that often looked like is that when we gave up sugar in
the past, our flour consumption gradually increased until it took
over our diets. This is because food addiction is both a *substance*
addiction and a *process* or behavioral addiction, meaning we are
addicted to the substance we put in our mouths, yes, but also to
the act of eating itself. These first two Bright Lines, eliminating
sugar and flour, get us sober from the substance component of
food addiction.

To begin the profound work of healing our bodies and minds,
we must get the addictive substances out of our systems. Once we
get clean and sober, only then can we finally get free.

ON THIS BRIGHT DAY,
I GLADLY EMBRACE MY FOOD PLAN
AS MY PATH TO FREEDOM.

MEALS

To lengthen thy life, lessen thy meals.
— BENJAMIN FRANKLIN

The average person decides 221 times per day whether and what to eat. That is 221 opportunities to take an action contrary to our goals. Before Bright Line Eating many of us grazed all day, eating at the table, in our cars, at our desks, in movie theatres and sports stadiums, on the couch, and in bed.

Having a Bright Line of only eating meals—never grazing or snacking—gives us the gift of now having fewer food decisions to make. Giving the body time after a meal to empty the stomach and digest before the next meal is going to be a new experience for many of us. And by not eating between meals, we will be able to transform much of our environment into a food-free place.

We start to think not just, "No, thank you; I don't eat sugar or flour," but "No, thank you; *I don't eat now*." By following through on these decisions in our set mealtime windows, life stops being a buffet. And we set ourselves up for success.

ON THIS BRIGHT DAY,

I WILL FULLY ENJOY MY COMMITTED MEALS AND NOTICE
THE CLARITY THEY BRING.

QUANTITIES

The lure of quantity is the most dangerous of all.
— SIMONE WEIL

Living with food addiction is exhausting. If we carry excess weight, we may feel physically fatigued from that burden. But there is also a mental exhaustion that comes from the endless negotiating around what we are going to eat. Weighing and measuring our food is the Bright Line that allows our brains to calm down and stop calculating: *Is this enough? Did I eat too much? Since I was light on fruit, maybe I could have more grains?* Those debates, questions, and suggestions quiet down when we put our food on the scale and measure the ounces precisely. And that freedom from food chatter is the biggest gift of Bright Line Eating.

Be patient with the process. For people who are used to eating and never feeling full, it will take some time and some artificial boundaries being imposed for your brain to understand what constitutes a healthy portion. Once you have been on Maintenance for a while, the Quantities Line is the one that is most likely to slip. Being precise about weighing and measuring is the way to tighten things up if you find yourself once again thinking too much about food. It is really not a triumph if our minds are still bargaining and obsessing. Give yourself the gift of absolute freedom.

ON THIS BRIGHT DAY,

I TAKE MY QUANTITIES BRIGHT LINE SERIOUSLY,
KNOWING IT IS SETTING ME FREE.

NMF

We are indeed much more than what we eat,
but what we eat can nevertheless help us to
be much more than what we are.

— ADELLE DAVIS

In our recovery journey we need to be able to talk about what we are saying "no" to. And because studies show that addicted brains are far more suspectable to cues like images and words, *Not My Food* (NMF) is the shorthand we use to signify anything that we did not commit to eating today. It could be food that contains sugar and flour, it could be food that is normally just fine in the food plan but was not what you chose ahead of time to eat, or it could be foods that other folks eat with no trouble but that give you difficulty.

We use the acronym NMF, rather than name specific foods, so that we don't trigger ourselves or others into thinking inordinately about an old favorite. And it prevents us from getting sucked into a rabbit hole of shared reminiscence of food that gave us a short-lived high but ultimately undermined our health goals and robbed us of the lives we wanted to be living. Calling something NMF in our heads removes all judgment and means that our family and friends can enjoy it, but it is simply not for us—not today.

ON THIS BRIGHT DAY,
I WILL RESPECT THAT THERE ARE FOODS
I DO NOT EAT AND GIVE GRATITUDE FOR THOSE I DO.

January 7

AUTOMATICITY

Habits mean we don't strain ourselves to make decisions,
weigh choices, dole out rewards, or prod ourselves to begin.
Life becomes simpler, and many daily hassles vanish.

— GRETCHEN RUBIN

We all have automaticity with a number of daily activities, such as grooming or driving. We need to cultivate that kind of automaticity in our meal preparation and food consumption as well, because once something becomes automatic, we don't have to use willpower to accomplish it and this frees up oceans of energy for other more meaningful tasks.

In service of that, look at where you can cultivate repetition. Maybe make sure your mealtimes become consistent. Maybe consider eating the same thing for several days in a row so that the preparation of a Bright meal becomes more automatic. Perhaps eat the same thing for breakfast every single day with small seasonal variations or adopt that approach for lunch and dinner as well, particularly at the beginning while you are laying down these new neural tracts.

The more attention and care you give at the beginning of this program, the sooner these actions will become automatic and the freer you will become. Give yourself the gift of repetition today to build the automaticity of tomorrow.

ON THIS BRIGHT DAY,

I WILL EMBRACE REPETITION AS THE FOUNDATION
OF MY FREEDOM.

HUNGER IS NOT AN EMERGENCY

> And she saw now that the strong impulses
> which had once wrecked her happiness were the forces
> that had enabled her to rebuild her life out of the ruins.
>
> — ELLEN GLASGOW

The process of getting sober from sugar and flour entails allowing many uncomfortable emotions and sensations to surface. Hunger is one of the most challenging because we may never have ignored it before. When you experience hunger, sometimes for the first time in ages, it can feel scary because it is so foreign. But learning to ride the wave of physical hunger becomes part of the work. It is truly a meditative practice. When you feel hunger, stop, notice, tune into the sensation, and breathe.

How does it actually feel? Is it a tightening? Is it a rumbling or butterfly feeling? Is it uncomfortable—or is it something else? Also give yourself the gift of noticing that, even if the next meal is hours away, the hunger passes. Especially if you can drink a big glass of water or get up and walk for a few minutes.

The fact is that for those of us who have come to food recovery in need of losing excess weight, that process requires some hunger. We make peace with that by knowing that we are getting enough food to function well, but not so much that we won't lose weight. Remembering that "hunger is not an emergency" is the mantra that helps us breathe through this—temporary—challenge.

ON THIS BRIGHT DAY,

I TRUST THAT MY NEEDS ARE GETTING MET.

BLE AND FAMILIES

Happiness is a sort of perfume. You can't pour it on somebody
else without getting a few drops on yourself.
— JAMES VAN DER ZEE

When it comes to making this huge lifestyle change, some of us may have supportive families, others may have indifferent families, and still others may have family members who feel threatened by our new habits. If you are feeling challenged, please know that most family members will eventually learn to honor your commitment and not sabotage your efforts. And those who eat with you often enjoy a healthier diet as well.

If your family is not as supportive as you would like, it is important to remember that you have made a shift that may be impacting them in ways they did not ask for or have a voice in. They might be mourning losing a buddy in their own addictive habits. It is not your job to change them; just work your program and let that be an inspiration. Be grateful for the accommodations they make *and* check to see if you have actually asked for what you need, including possibly keeping some NMF out of sight.

Even if your family never comes around, know that the Bright Line Eating community will come to feel like an incredibly warm and connected surrogate family that will provide deep social support on every step of your Bright Journey.

ON THIS BRIGHT DAY,

I OFFER MY BEST TO MY LOVING FAMILY AND
ENJOY THE SUPPORT THEY CAN OFFER.

January 10

NMD

Drink does not drown care, but waters it,
and makes it grow faster.
— BENJAMIN FRANKLIN

Just as we use NMF to denote foods that are off our plan, we use the term NMD to describe beverages we do not drink, which include anything alcoholic or artificially sweetened. Abstaining from alcohol may not be a struggle for some but could be more challenging for others, such as those who have forged a strong social link between alcohol and entertaining or fellowship.

Hard alcohols are called spirits, and people are often looking to enhance their perceived reality through alcohol consumption. But we can find a sense of raised spirit or spiritual connection without altering our brain chemistry. Learning to enjoy these connections without specific beverages is part of the growth in our BLE experiences. Once we learn to do that, it can be a real blessing to live life without alcohol and find more authentic, more powerful ways of connecting to others, ourselves, and the universe.

ON THIS BRIGHT DAY,

I WILL LOOK BEYOND ALCOHOL TO FOSTER
MEANINGFUL CONNECTION.

January 11

SUPPORT

Proximity was their support;
like walls after an earthquake they could fall no further
for they had fallen against each other.
— ELIZABETH BOWEN

Humans are herd animals. Several thousand years ago, none of us would have survived without a community, and still today our brains prioritize belonging. Behaviors that threaten our sense of belonging will be rapidly shed and traded for behaviors that are approved of in the tight-knit groups that we belong to. For this reason, we find that people who stick with Bright Line Eating long term and experience the full Bright Transformation are the ones who have found tight-knit groups within their newfound food community.

While friends and family may be supportive, it is key to get support from others who are following the Bright Lines because they understand the unique challenges and triumphs of living Bright. Find support in the online communities, post and respond daily, reach out to those who live in your area, find a Buddy to contact regularly, and perhaps get a temporary Guide if you need more help. Most of us do not ask for what we need often enough. But in the BLE community, we welcome being asked to provide support and we applaud ourselves when we ask for it. This is a road we walk arm in arm.

ON THIS BRIGHT DAY,

I RECEIVE AND GIVE THE VITAL GIFT OF SUPPORT.

THE BRIGHT BODY

People who identify themselves with their body
often find the latter half of life a great burden.
Only when you learn to identify yourself with the Self will
the latter half of your life become a great blessing.

— EKNATH EASWARAN

It is easy to have an unrealistic image of what our bodies should be in an economy that relies on telling us that our bodies are nothing more than projects that forever need expensive fixes. That puts unattainable perfection forever out of reach. Learning to see ourselves realistically, especially after losing weight, is a process. Rather than attending to an image in the mirror, consider working internally to determine what your Bright Body will be able to *do* rather than what it will look like. What kind of physical tasks would you love to do in your Bright Body? Hike the Camino de Santiago? Ride bikes with your grandchildren? Do a chin-up?

By focusing on how you would like to move and feel in your body, you reclaim your joy and learn to inhabit your skin with an ease and comfort that is beautiful and attractive no matter your size. And the sooner you happily inhabit your body, the more joyful your journey will be.

ON THIS BRIGHT DAY,

I WILL POUR LOVE AND GRATITUDE INTO MY BODY
FOR ALL IT CAN DO.

January 13
INNER REBEL

There is no coming to consciousness without pain.
— CARL JUNG

A lot of us developed a strong Rebel inner part whose job it was to protect us from pain in our childhood. Now we can discover that our Rebel inner part pushes back against Bright Line Eating as if there is some authority figure demanding that we work this program. It is helpful to reassure that part of ourselves that we are choosing this plan freely, that there is no Bright Line police, and that there is no judgment coming from the program about what we do or don't do on our journey. We are free to adopt whatever aspects of Bright Line Eating work for us and relinquish whatever parts of the program do not. Moreover, that Rebel inner part can be given a new role: a rabble-rouser against the "normal" way of eating that society has adopted that is leading so many people to die too young and in pain. A Rebel does their own thing and there is no more powerful stance against the indulgence of processed food culture than food sobriety.

ON THIS BRIGHT DAY,
I GET TO KNOW MY INNER PARTS BETTER
WITH GRATITUDE AND CURIOSITY.

January 14
HABITS

Success is the product of daily habits—
not once-in-a-lifetime transformations.
— JAMES CLEAR

Many of us come to Bright Line Eating with deeply entrenched habits around our eating. Some stun us once we start to pay attention to them. Perhaps you have to uncouple watching TV and eating NMF, or release the habit of stopping at the same drive-through every day. The best way to rid yourself of a bad habit is to develop a better habit in its place.

In Bright Line Eating the consistent repetition of tiny daily actions creates our flow. We start with our food. At first it takes a long time to study the food plan and figure out what we're going to eat. Eventually we get into a rhythm where planning out our food for the next day just takes a few moments.

At first breaking unhealthy food habits may feel overwhelming, but that's because we are bringing our behaviors to the level of consciousness where we can examine them and do things differently over time. Eventually, our new right way of eating and living will feel automatic and the food will fade into the background. That is the beauty of habits.

ON THIS BRIGHT DAY,

I WILL EMBRACE THE GIFT OF NEW HABITS.

SUSCEPTIBILITY SCORE

*What you have become is the price you paid
to get what you used to want.*
— MIGNON MCLAUGHLIN

When we begin our recovery journey in Bright Line Eating, we take the Food Addiction Susceptibility Quiz, which reveals how vulnerable we are to the pull of refined food. This is invaluable information to have. If we have been bingeing or eating wildly for years, knowing our score can relieve us from any shame or misguided notion that we are deficient in willpower or moral fiber. If we are high on the Susceptibility Scale, we know that we cannot safely ingest flour or sugar without it triggering cravings.

But what if we are lower on the scale? What good does it do to know that? BLE works for those of us who are low on the Susceptibility Scale as well, especially if we have weight to lose and feel drawn to a structured way of eating to solve that problem. We will modify the plan as needed and use the Bright Lines as guides to get the results we want.

The joy is that once there is a diagnosis, there is a potential plan of treatment—our own personal Bright Roadmap. If you have not yet taken the brief quiz to determine how susceptible your brain is to the pull of addictive foods, please do so at FoodAddictionQuiz.com. Knowledge is power.

ON THIS BRIGHT DAY,

I WELCOME THE TRUTH ABOUT WHAT I CAN
AND CANNOT EAT SAFELY.

HEALING THE BRAIN

The boredom produced by a complete absence
of risk is . . . a sickness of the soul.
— SIMONE WEIL

Neurotransmitters like serotonin and oxytocin help us to feel satisfied and grateful in the here and now. Dopamine is the only neurotransmitter that orients toward the future, that allows us to imagine a world that does not exist in this moment. It is also the neurotransmitter of dissatisfaction. It propels us toward wanting more and better, but by its very definition, is never satiated. Because sugar and flour provide a spike in dopamine, when we stop eating the foods that brought us that quick hit, there will be a sense of loss, sadness, and perhaps even bleakness. But it is temporary.

We can weather the restlessness, hopelessness, despair, or mild anxiety with the support of our community who have walked this path before us. Because our brains *do* heal, the sun will break through the clouds, and we will take even greater pleasure than ever before in ordinary things. And we will see and process them through a sparkly Bright brain.

Let the community carry you as you heal.

ON THIS BRIGHT DAY,

I RIDE THE WAVES OF HEALING WITH
GRATITUDE AND GRACE.

IDENTITY SHIFT

He allowed himself to be swayed by his conviction
that human beings are not born once and for all on the day
their mothers give birth to them, but that life obliges them
over and over again to give birth to themselves.
— GABRIEL GARCÍA MÁRQUEZ

Because so many of us have dieted for so much of our lives, it may be challenging to think of BLE as a way of eating for life. When people start, they often simply cannot imagine a lifetime without eating sugar and flour. But those who have been living Bright for years absolutely can.

Over time a big identity shift will take place. We build it brick by brick, Bright meal by Bright meal, one day at a time. We build it by writing down our food the night before, then the next day eating only and exactly that.

As the identity of a person who doesn't eat sugar or flour and doesn't eat between meals takes hold, saying no to daily invitations becomes the norm. As the identity of a person who seeks and gives support on this journey takes hold, we become a supported and supportive person. By watching ourselves perform those actions consistently, we become the person who does this. We become who we are at the *deepest* level: Bright.

ON THIS BRIGHT DAY,

I TAKE MANY SMALL ACTIONS TO BUILD MY NEW IDENTITY.

January 18
TRAVEL

Sooner or later, we must realize there is no station,
no one place to arrive at once and for all.
The true joy of life is the trip.
— ROBERT J. HASTINGS

If the goal of our recovery journey is to be reborn, then we must think of the beginning of our journey as a cocoon or chrysalis, a place to which we retreat to do the transformational work required of us. A place where we control the environment and can mitigate the challenges our fledgling sobriety will face.

For this reason, try to avoid traveling at the beginning of your journey. The stress of unpredictability and the seduction of eating out meal after meal can reawaken your dopamine receptors and leave you vulnerable in a place where you may feel cut off from support.

If you must venture forth, plan ahead, research menus, commit as many meals ahead of time as possible, bring a small food scale, and even consider bringing your food with you. With preparation and forethought, any journey can be a Bright Journey, but it will require a deeper level of commitment and intense support. With both—and in time—you will be that soaring butterfly in any situation or location.

ON THIS BRIGHT DAY,
I TRAVEL WITH MY BLE PROGRAM AND AM OPEN,
CURIOUS, AND SAFE WHEREVER I AM.

LONELINESS

---

*We have all known the long loneliness and
we have learned that the only solution is love and
that love comes with community.*
— DOROTHY DAY

Has food been a constant companion? Even a best friend? Putting our food on a scale and limiting it to three meals a day can leave what feels like a hole in our lives. Maybe you can't even identify it as loneliness because you have always eaten something the moment that feeling arose.

In the early days of BLE, we learn to lean into that loneliness, feel the emptiness, and discover that it won't kill us. In fact, it is here to let us know it is time to explore greater connection. With others by picking up the phone. With yourself by journaling, meditating, or starting a practice like yoga to help you feel more embodied. With a higher power through prayer, meditation, or simply being in nature. Ask someone out for a tea after a class or a hike to connect inwardly and outwardly. There is so much connection available to you on your journey. You do not need to walk it alone.

ON THIS BRIGHT DAY,

IF I DO NOT FEEL LONELY, I WILL REACH
OUT TO SOMEONE WHO MAY.

NO MAGIC FORMULA

But I choose to let the mystery be.
— IRIS DEMENT

It may be tempting to see Bright Line Eating as magic if you have spent your life looking for the perfect diet, book, workshop, or recipe that will help you lose weight and keep it off, only to discover that total food sobriety is far more effective than anything you have ever tried. But BLE is only effective if we keep doing it wholly and fully. It is a holistic program with many strands that weave a powerful net to hold you, and it is important to use as many tools and enter as many parts of the community as you need to keep your Lines Bright. The proof is always in your Lines—if they are wobbly or wonky, you need to work a stronger program. No one habit or tool will be the one and only thing to do the trick, so keep leaning into all the available resources and let the integrated system of support lift you.

ON THIS BRIGHT DAY,

I EXPLORE NEW ASPECTS OF THE PROGRAM.

GRATITUDE

A thankful person is thankful under all circumstances. A complaining soul complains even if they live in paradise.

— BAHA'U'LLAH

Cicero said gratitude is "not only the greatest of the virtues, but the parent of all of the others," and studies show that gratitude literally changes our brain. While there can be days in the weight-loss phase that can feel so hard it does not seem like there is anything to be grateful for, cultivating a discipline of appreciating something or someone before each meal will transform you on the inside.

If you have an area of your life that is especially troublesome, write a gratitude list for it. Repeating that practice over a series of days can shift your perspective on any situation, and maybe even shift the situation itself. Find a way to establish a habit of gratitude, whether it is a list you write down, a video or text you send to a group, or a quiet reflection first thing in the morning. You will be setting an intention to look all day long for what is working in your life, and that in itself is Bright living.

ON THIS BRIGHT DAY,

I FIND GRATITUDE FOR MY CHALLENGES.

January 22
SILENCE

In the attitude of silence the soul finds the path in a clearer light,
and what is elusive and deceptive resolves itself into
crystal clearness.

— MAHATMA GANDHI

One of the great gifts of eating the Bright Line way is the quiet we get in our heads after our brains begin to heal. When we make the decision to eat only and exactly what we have written down the night before, so long as we keep putting our food on the scale one day at a time, we do not have to debate every piece of NMF that crosses our path. That inner silence leaves space for new ideas, subtle awareness, and deepening peace that replenishes us in ways we hoped food might when we were eating too much. Our minds settle down. It all gets clearer. And we notice moments of spaciousness and begin to develop a beautiful relationship with silence.

ON THIS BRIGHT DAY,
I WILL RETURN TO THE PEACE WITHIN.

OBLIGATION OR GUIDANCE

Each time you set a healthy boundary,
you say "yes" to more freedom.
— NANCY LEVIN

Notice how many actions you take each day that feel like obligations. Sometimes, of course, we have responsibilities and commitments we do not feel like following through on, but we must. Or we have tasks that keep our lives functional. But how many times do we simply go through the motions on something because we think we have to? How often do we give ourselves the gift of unstructured time to listen to what we want to do next? To connect with our deep inner guidance? Living without the compulsion to eat NMF affords us the opportunity to listen more deeply to our inner selves. It is often said in food recovery that we keep our food black and white so we can experience life in vibrant color, meaning when our food is in its place, there is a lot of room to explore options. How might you explore your options today?

ON THIS BRIGHT DAY,

I TAKE EXTRA TIME TO LISTEN DEEPLY
AND TAKE ACTION ON THE GUIDANCE
THAT COMES FROM WITHIN.

January 24
ONLY CONNECT

Addictions represent finite answers to infinite
longings. But adding up the finite over and over
will never equal the infinite.
— TIMOTHY MCMAHAN KING

Most addicts require connection to recover. That is all most of us were seeking in food—connection with ourselves in a comfortable way, connection with others using food to bond and celebrate, and connection with something larger through the sublimity of that first bite. But food is a poor proxy for connection.

When we experience our Bright Transformation, we get the real joy of truly connecting with ourselves, knowing that we are doing right by our whole selves. Then we start to form deeper and more satisfying bonds with others because we are more present in the moment with them. Through the doorway of that present moment is the miracle of connection.

ON THIS BRIGHT DAY,

I WALK TOWARD OTHERS WITH AN OPEN HEART, KNOWING
THAT CONNECTION IS WHAT I AM TRULY HUNGRY FOR.

January 25
SERVICE

There is nothing to make you like other human beings
so much as doing things for them.
— ZORA NEALE HURSTON

The simplest formula for sustaining a Bright Transformation for decades upon decades is focusing on gratitude and service to solidify any recovery program. A one-third, one-third, one-third approach to connection can be helpful.

We spend one-third of our connection time fostering bonds with people who are supporting us on our journey—people who have wisdom to share because they have traveled the road before us. We spend one-third of that time connecting with people who are at the same place we are—people who feel like peers, our "littermates," if you will. And then we spend one-third of our connection time being of service to others who are struggling or newer on their journey. That might mean taking their food commitment every day. If we are already in Maintenance, it might mean supporting someone else who is landing their weight-loss plane. When we need support, knowing that we are all interdependent as we walk this path will ground us. After the myopia of addiction, service is something that we must reorient ourselves toward—and the rewards are boundless.

ON THIS BRIGHT DAY,

I TRAVEL IN AN INTERDEPENDENT NETWORK OF SUPPORT.

ON THE CUSP

Character cannot be developed in ease and quiet.
Only through experience of trial and suffering can the soul
be strengthened, vision cleared, ambition inspired,
and success achieved.

— HELEN KELLER

Being on the cusp of change can feel like being on the edge of the pool before diving in or on the outside of the jump rope before entering the game. Just as children beginning a growth spurt may get cranky, we may also find that we now have resistance where we once were willing. That resistance is a powerful internal indicator that it is time to shift into curiosity about what is going on and what will help us break through to the next level. Our inner Rebel often knows we are on the cusp before we are conscious of it and may kick up objections that don't make sense or might keep us from the growth we need. This is the key moment to surrender yet again to a deeper way of living in the world and to not delay in taking whatever action is suggested for your next step.

ON THIS BRIGHT DAY,

I WILL NOTICE MY RESISTANCE AND BE WILLING TO
EMBRACE THE NEXT CHANGE.

PUTTING DOWN ROOTS

Plants bear witness to the reality of roots.
— MOSES MAIMONIDES

Sometimes even happiness can feel destabilizing. If we have become accustomed to using food to ground ourselves when good things happen (for fear we might metaphorically float away), we must find new ways of receiving the good we are creating in our lives.

When you are recovering from an addiction to always chasing that next hit of dopamine, it is important to put down roots in the moments of ease and joy, as subtle as they may be, so that they become the new set point for your emotions. Look inward—take a deep breath, sing, move your body, or dance. Then look outward, taking a mental picture of the beauty and sitting still with the feeling of contentment or success. You can literally expand your cellular capacity to experience joy by anchoring in the moment of awareness that, *Oh yes, this is what freedom feels like!*

ON THIS BRIGHT DAY,

I PUT THE ROOT OF MY RECOVERY DEEPER
INTO THE SOIL OF MY RECOVERY AND
CELEBRATE THE BLOSSOMS OF JOY
AND PEACE THAT EMERGE.

INVENTORIES

You cannot weave truth on a loom of lies.
— SUZETTE HADEN ELGIN

Over the years of addictive eating, we can develop the habit of not looking too closely—at our bodies or our choices. But now we must develop the opposite practice. Just as an airline pilot has a checklist of activities to do before taking off, no matter how long she has been flying, we need ways to inventory the various habits and tools we are using to become automatic in Bright Line Eating. What we measure we value, so honoring how our day went through a nightly inventory of what we did or did not do becomes an analytic tool to help us understand what we need more or less of in our life to keep our Lines Bright.

We use checklists in a variety of formats to measure what we need to keep an eye on. Where are we experiencing resistance? Is there a part of our program that needs tightening? Taking the time to check in, either on paper or digitally, gives us valuable information that we receive without judgment and accordingly take action on. We do not need to be afraid to look closely anymore.

ON THIS BRIGHT DAY,

I TAKE STOCK OF THE ACTIONS THAT HELP
KEEP MY LINES BRIGHT.

January 29
ACCEPTANCE

My happiness grows in direct proportion
to my acceptance, and in inverse
proportion to my expectations.
— MICHAEL J. FOX

There is a flow to life that is larger than any individual, and being in tune with it can make things much easier than trying to "push the river," as the ancient teachings say. Many of us come to food recovery accustomed to trying to control and manage our weight, our food, our lives, and even—perhaps especially—our family members and the people around us. And it can be very hard for us to now trust and surrender to the natural flow of the day. We want to rush to goal weight, to the end of cravings, to an imaginary finish line instead of accepting where we are and allowing each stage to teach us something valuable about ourselves and our journey.

ON THIS BRIGHT DAY,
I WILL FLOW WITH EVENTS AS THEY UNFOLD
AND TRUST ALL ELSE TO TAKE CARE OF ITSELF.

January 30
LOVING IT ALL

I accept the universe!
— MARGARET FULLER

The more you can love every aspect of maintaining your Bright Lines, the easier it becomes and the more your habits, tools, and connections will give you the deep nurturance you once may have sought from food. There is nothing sustainable about resenting having to weigh your food, or make recovery phone calls, or meditate in the mornings. If this notion of resentment persists, it can be helpful to stay relaxed, open, and curious about the Rebel inner part of you that perhaps doesn't love certain aspects of living a structured life that it sees as too rigid.

Exploring our resistance always takes our acceptance to the next level. If you can love the process and how each action you take is contributing to your well-being, then you are already there, regardless of what the scale may say. In other words, allowing yourself to love every aspect of your recovery, including the challenging or annoying parts, will transform you inside just as following your Bright Lines will transform your body.

ON THIS BRIGHT DAY,
I WILL ACTIVELY LOVE WHATEVER CROSSES MY PATH.

EMERGENCY ACTION PLAN

If you are tired, keep going. If you are scared, keep going.
If you are hungry, keep going.
If you want to taste freedom, keep going.
— HARRIET TUBMAN

On this journey we all face emergencies from time to time—a situation where we are so overwhelmed by some combination of emotions, stress, and seductive NMF that we sense that our sobriety is in imminent danger. The Emergency Action Plan (EAP) is a document tailor-made for that moment when we are not just struggling but feeling ourselves going under. (See Resources on page 383.)

Create your EAP from a place of ease and confidence, imagining yourself in potentially stressful, destabilizing situations and planning exactly what you will do in each of them. *If I am faced with X, I will immediately do Y.* Decide what actions you will need to take, whether simple or elaborate. Include some ways to reach out for help, distract yourself from negative thoughts, and build in a pause before acting on a craving.

"Breathe, Pray, Call" can be something you memorize and bring to mind at the first sign of a waver in your Bright Lines. Or you can have a series of steps, such as stretch, make a phone call, read something inspirational, and reach out for support online. Write out your EAP, carry it on your person, and memorize it. It can save your program.

ON THIS BRIGHT DAY,
I WILL PLAN AHEAD TO WEATHER
CHALLENGES IN THE FUTURE.

February

CALL BEFORE TAKING THE ADDICTIVE BITE

The one with the primary responsibility to the individual's future is that individual.

— DORCAS HARDY

There is a maxim in food recovery programs about picking up the phone before picking up the food. If you can create an Emergency Action Plan that includes calling until you get someone live, you will have built a barrier between the idea of NMF and the action of consuming it. This will only happen, however, if you are in the practice of calling people when life is smooth and you are not tempted to eat off plan.

When we first received the suggestion to make daily phone calls, some of us hated it and fought it with great resistance, but those who tried it found that the daily connection truly did revolutionize their experience, not just of doing Bright Line Eating, but of living life. It fills our spirits to be connected and have friends on this journey.

Practice today by calling someone, regardless of whether you are tempted to eat off plan. Having that in place will make it a familiar move to pick up the phone and share how vulnerable you are when crisis strikes.

ON THIS BRIGHT DAY,
I WILL PICK UP THE PHONE AND CONNECT
WITH A FELLOW TRAVELER ON THIS PATH.

KEEP YOUR EYES ON YOUR OWN PLATE

I thought I could change the world. It took me a hundred
years to figure out I can't change the world. I can
only change Bessie. And honey, that ain't easy either.

— A. ELIZABETH DELANY

The best we can hope to be in life is an example of love, compassion, and unconditional acceptance. Which is why we have a saying in Bright Line Eating: Keep your eyes on your own plate. Once we are on solid ground with our food sobriety and are doing well with our health and weight, it can be tempting to start judging other people's food choices. We may even want to help the people around us with how they live, how they behave, and how they show up in the world. But that can really be less about helping and more about controlling, directing, and managing others. The truth is, despite our good intentions, we are often the person least able to help a loved one with their food or weight. And the nudge to judge simply distances us from our loved ones and distracts us from what we should be focused on next.

Instead of commenting or internally criticizing someone else, the best practice is to stay focused on keeping our own Lines Bright and doing any inner work that may be calling.

ON THIS BRIGHT DAY,

I BRING MY ATTENTION BACK TO MYSELF
WHENEVER I FEEL JUDGMENT OF OTHERS.

February 3

ACCOUNTABILITY

Power can be taken, but not given.
The process of the taking is empowerment in itself.
— GLORIA STEINEM

It can be hard to shift to a system of accountability when for so many years many of us kept our food habits tucked away in shame. But without external accountability—someone we commit our food and habits to—many of us find that we cut corners and eventually lose our Bright Lines. Having accountability outside ourselves relieves us from relying on willpower to succeed and provides the support and externalized structure we know we truly need to work the program.

At the beginning, that kind of structure can be the difference between sticking with the program or not. Later, many of us find that having external accountability is beneficial as we transition to Maintenance. And it is invaluable if you find your Lines are getting wobbly. But you need to find an accountability structure that works for you. You will know it is working because you will feel beholden, and your Lines will be Bright and sparkly.

ON THIS BRIGHT DAY,

I WILL ALIGN MY POWER WITH ANOTHER'S TO DO
WHAT I HAVE NOT DONE BEFORE.

NON-SCALE VICTORIES

> If you believe in yourself and have dedication
> and pride and never quit, you'll be a winner.
> The price of victory is high but so are the rewards.
> — BEAR BRYANT

Rather than staying hyperfocused on losing weight, BLE invites you to notice all the other blessings that emerge when you live Bright. We come to know peace of mind, more authentic connections with others, ease of movement, and growing confidence. Keeping track of these "Non-Scale Victories" (NSVs) can replenish your willpower during challenging times and help maintain your focus when keeping your Lines Bright becomes routine.

By developing the habit of tuning in to these other changes, which are often subtle, you will develop a perspective that will sustain your momentum and keep you going when weight loss stalls, or when you reach Maintenance and no longer have weight-loss victories to look forward to. Non-Scale Victories might include not being tempted by samples at the grocery store or noticing you are more interested in people than food. Some people accomplish major career shifts and powerful new directions in their lives, whether it is ending an unhealthy relationship or moving somewhere that feels more like home. The real benefits of food sobriety simply cannot be measured by a bathroom scale.

ON THIS BRIGHT DAY,

I PROUDLY NOTICE AND CLAIM ALL THE THINGS THAT HAVE
IMPROVED SINCE I CHOSE TO BEGIN THIS WAY OF LIFE.

SLEEP

Sleep is the best meditation.
— DALAI LAMA

Most adults do not get enough sleep, and there is a growing body of research indicating it is *the* foundational practice for physical and mental health as well as longevity. In our Bright world, nourishing sleep helps us rebuild the mental and emotional buffer we need to navigate our weight-loss journey. And it is during sleep that our bodies clear the toxins our shrinking fat cells are releasing into our bloodstream.

Sleep helps us live Bright, and living Bright also helps our sleep. When we only eat three times a day at set mealtimes, we align the external circadian clocks in our digestive organs with our central circadian clock in our hypothalamus, and as a result, our circadian rhythm gets stronger and our sleep vastly improves. With our blood sugar regulated and our days structured, we give ourselves the opportunity to follow basic sleep hygiene practices with a consistency that may have always been out of reach for us.

Bedtime becomes an evening routine that nourishes the soul: we put away our screens an hour before bedtime, release stress from the day through journaling or meditating, and give ourselves something soothing or relaxing to listen to, read, or experience. Bedtime becomes a gift.

ON THIS BRIGHT DAY,
I CELEBRATE HOW MY SLEEP IS IMPROVING
AND ENJOY FEELING RESTORED.

BUDDY

> All sorrows can be borne if you put them
> into a story or tell a story about them.
> — ISAK DINESEN

Many participants in Bright Line Eating have a Buddy whom they contact daily. The ideal Buddy is someone who comes to know you well—not only your food plan and history with BLE, but also the ups and downs of your daily life. Research on Bright Line Eating has demonstrated that after just a couple of months in the program, people feel more supported and connected in the world. That benefit goes deep and pervades all aspects of their lives, from their sense of happiness and well-being to their health.

Our support circle goes beyond food—it is about living a richer, more meaningful life. As we walk the Bright path, we find our connections with others become deeper and more fulfilling, and that can all start with a single Buddy we talk to at the same time each day or text regularly—someone who becomes a friend. We develop individual friendships, and before long, we are surrounded by a sustainable, life-giving network of support.

ON THIS BRIGHT DAY,

I WILL REACH OUT WITH AN OPEN HEART.

ALLOW SUCCESS

*If everyone is moving forward together,
then success takes care of itself.*
— HENRY FORD

During a BLE journey, many of us experience levels of success in weight loss that we never have before. This can be a heady experience, destabilizing even, because often we find that we are as afraid of success as we are of failure. Success can be daunting. Allowing success means taking in that you deserve to feel good in your body.

You deserve to get this excess weight off. You deserve to be free of cravings. You deserve to come back into balance. And you deserve to share it with others, both because it inspires them and because it helps you claim your success. Set aside time to celebrate the milestones you reach, both in terms of the scale and in other areas of your life, in order to increase your capacity to experience and savor success. The beautiful thing is that if you stick with it, over time you will absolutely become accustomed to the feeling of success—which will allow even more success into your life. And it can start here.

ON THIS BRIGHT DAY,

I SAVOR MY SUCCESSES.

SOFT FOCUS

Who looks outside, dreams;
who looks inside, awakes.
— CARL JUNG

When we were in the throes of addiction, NMF got all our focus. We thought about it, hunted it down, and consumed it with relentless ferocity. In the places where it was on offer, our senses were heightened as we took in the promise of each package, each menu description, each ingredient as though we could get high just by reading a label or touching a menu. We were crawling out of ourselves with anticipation.

A new way to move through those same aisles and restaurants is to let them blur. As you enter the store or restaurant or party, pull your focus inward, into the centered part of yourself, the core that is in balance and harmony without NMF or NMD. Allow your surroundings to go into soft focus, a brightly colored abstract painting you are walking past on your way to your rainbow of vegetables. Imagine the tentacles of your attention retracting until they envelop you, your heart, and your soul. Go within and your Bright program will be your refuge.

ON THIS BRIGHT DAY,
I ALLOW THE WORLD OF TEMPTATION
TO BLUR AS I LOOK INWARD.

February 9

EXERCISE?

To everything there is a season,
a time for every purpose under heaven.
— ECCLESIASTES 3:1

BLE differs from many weight-loss programs in that we avoid starting a vigorous exercise regimen in the early days. Too much willpower can be diverted into exercise, and we fall prey to the compensation effect where we justify extra food because we are hungrier and think we have earned it by burning calories. The math doesn't work out that way, so we focus instead on using the tools available to us in BLE.

We put our energy and willpower toward sticking to our Bright Lines, and we establish a solid foundation that will eventually afford us the luxury of exercising. Once we are stable in our Bright Lines, or perhaps when we have transitioned to Maintenance, it is time to get active, and we can focus on automaticity and building exercise into our morning habit stack. We can use a lot of the lessons that work for us with Bright Line Eating to get into exercise. It doesn't take much. And it is important.

Because research shows that while exercise does not help us lose weight, it definitely helps us maintain our Bright Body once we have had our transformation. And there is hardly a greater joy in life than exercising in a Bright Body.

ON THIS BRIGHT DAY,

I WILL MOVE ACCORDING TO THE WISDOM
OF WHERE I AM ON MY BLE JOURNEY.

POSITIVITY

In a kind of paradoxical way, it is how we face all
of the things that seem to be negative in our lives that
determines the kind of person we become.

— ARCHBISHOP DESMOND TUTU

Our brains come hardwired with a negativity bias. Thousands of years ago they evolved to always be scanning the environment for threats, assessing what is wrong and what needs to be improved. Early humans with a carefree attitude did not survive to pass on their genes. But today, with our basic needs hopefully mostly provided for (and fewer saber-toothed tigers on our commute), this negativity bias does not serve us well. And alas, an extra-strong dose of negativity bias is part of addiction.

When our thinking grows more negative, critical, or harsh, it is usually a sign that it is time to shore up our program. Happiness and positive thinking are facilitated by healthy eating and can be strengthened by developing a discipline of appreciation, positive affirmations, and a focus on what is working. Cultivating a positivity bias can be a beautiful way to live.

ON THIS BRIGHT DAY,
I WILL IMAGINE A GENEROUS AND POSITIVE
INTERPRETATION OF OTHERS' ACTIONS.

COME ALL THE WAY IN, SIT ALL THE WAY DOWN

Wholehearted living is not a onetime choice. It is a process.
In fact, I believe it's the journey of a lifetime.
— BRENÉ BROWN

If you are just beginning BLE, this is a perfect opportunity to place yourself in the center of the community, say yes to every invitation, and use all the tools provided. That kind of wholehearted approach will establish a great foundation for living Bright the rest of your life.

Cutting corners, which many of us were prone to do, can erode your success and slow your momentum. If you find yourself hesitant to connect with others in the program, use a certain tool, or let go of a specific food, get curious about the story you are telling yourself about belonging.

Perhaps it is time to challenge yourself with a new practice of taking a deep breath and picking a chair on the inside of the BLE community. We want you close! After all, no one ever falls off the middle of the wagon.

ON THIS BRIGHT DAY,
I WILL NOTICE WHERE I AM HOLDING BACK.
I WILL CHOOSE TO GIVE MY WHOLE SELF
TO THIS PROGRAM, JUST FOR TODAY.

HAPPINESS

Happiness consists more in the small conveniences or pleasures that occur every day, than in great pieces of good fortune that happen but seldom in the course of a life.

— BENJAMIN FRANKLIN

Happiness, they say, is an "inside job." What this means in BLE is that our happiness cannot be dependent on a number on the scale, the behavior of another person, or even the deliciousness of our food. We are looking for a deeper form of happiness that comes from living in integrity, following through on our word, and allowing ourselves to be known.

The actions that bring about happiness may appear mundane and ordinary, but they add up to a life well lived. For some of us, our food is foundational to our level of happiness, meaning it is the one thing that needs to be in place for everything else to feel right. When our food is off, no matter how great our circumstances might be on the outside, we do not feel happy. And when our food is on track, no matter how terrible our circumstances, we have the deep faith that everything is going to be okay.

If you notice that you are sabotaging other areas of your life as you lose weight, you may want to get a bigger container to hold your happiness. That usually means more contact in quiet time with your innermost self, more connection to others who can celebrate with you, and an attitude shift that the sky's the limit for your life.

ON THIS BRIGHT DAY,

I RECOGNIZE EVEN THE SMALLEST MOMENTS OF HAPPINESS.

DIET MENTALITY VS. IDENTITY

I'm sick and tired of being sick and tired.

— FANNIE LOU HAMER

It is understandable to have remnants of diet mentality, to conceive of the BLE food plan as something temporary that can be discarded when you reach your goal weight or because of a special occasion. But that is not the foundation of sustainable change.

Pay attention: Are sugar and flour foods you "can't" eat rather than "don't" eat? Do you have "good" and "bad" days depending on how Bright your Lines are? You can tell the people who nurture a strong Bright Identity because they are not focused on a number on the scale. They have settled in. This is the way they do their food. So, it does not really matter how quickly or slowly their weight melts off.

The shift from "doing" Bright Line Eating to "being" a Bright Line Eater likely will not occur overnight, because identity is built meal by meal, day by day. You will gradually step into a more fully realized identity as a Bright Line Eater the more consistently you follow the plan. Also, dieting is typically done by individuals. Identity is formed in community. Stay in the BLE community to achieve deep change.

ON THIS BRIGHT DAY,

I WILL FOCUS ON IDENTITY AND COMMUNITY.

February 14
LOVE

You want to be loved because you do not love;
but the moment you love, it is finished, you are no longer
inquiring whether or not somebody loves you.

— J. KRISHNAMURTI

Today is devoted to romantic love and often connected to NMF. BLE works to uncouple the two and reinforce the importance of *self*-love and treating others lovingly. Working the Bright Line Eating program, one meal and one action at a time, is a demonstration of care for ourselves that grows into a very deep form of self-love.

When it comes to others, people often comment on the loving support they receive in Bright Line Eating. We take great care to set a tone of kindness and tolerance rather than criticism or even advice-giving. Nobody changes because they have been judged; we change because we have been loved exactly as we are and invited to be our best selves. Offering yourself loving compassion as you undertake this BLE journey can be the greatest gift of all—the weight loss is a bonus. When we love ourselves, we eat better, move more, listen to what our heart desires, say no to things that are not helpful or necessary, and offer the same to everyone we encounter.

ON THIS BRIGHT DAY,

I WILL SHOW MYSELF LOVE THROUGH MY FOOD CHOICES.

PIERCING PERFECTION

*The highest form of human intelligence is
to observe yourself without judgment.*
— J. KRISHNAMURTI

Many of us come into the program with a Food Controller inner part that has developed a lot of perfectionism, which stems from a well-founded fear that, if given an inch, the Food Indulger part of us will take a mile. Which leads to a fear of failure, a fear of allowing any deviation whatsoever creep in because in the past it has all unraveled in front of our eyes. But learning to let something be imperfect without having to sabotage the whole endeavor is such an important skill. And for many of us, even reading something like that feels threatening because it seems so important to keep our Lines Bright 100 percent.

But while it is important to follow the Bright Lines 100 percent, there are many times when the habits that buoy us slip, and learning to acknowledge and adjust without judgment becomes an important skill. Not having a stellar meditation routine, neglecting the Nightly Checklist, or not keeping up with phone calls during a busy time can provide an opportunity to not be perfectionistic about every aspect of our lives.

Keeping your Lines perfectly is more about being in recovery than perfectionism.

ON THIS BRIGHT DAY,

I NOTICE WHAT I AM DOING, WHAT I AM RESISTING,
AND WHAT I HAVE NEGLECTED IN MY BLE
PROGRAM WITHOUT JUDGMENT.

ENCOURAGING SIGNS

True progress is never made by spasms.
Real progress is growth. It must begin in the seed.

— ANNA JULIA COOPER

Sometimes when the weight loss stalls or Maintenance becomes mundane, we can get discouraged and look to our old ways for excitement—NMF and NMD. But there is a better way, albeit uncharted territory. And that is to notice the signs of progress, however small.

Take a moment to revel in what is working and acknowledge everything you have achieved. Did you pass the break room without even thinking about the snacks on the table? Have you had a great stretch of making support calls every day? Did you perform some physical task with ease? Those are all wonderful markers on this road.

What we focus on expands in our consciousness, and then our brain finds evidence of whatever hypothesis we are trying out. So why not put your time and energy into signs of improved health and happiness?

ON THIS BRIGHT DAY,

I NOTICE GROWTH AND APPRECIATE ANY AND
ALL FORWARD MOMENTUM.

MILESTONES AND CELEBRATIONS

Nothing ever comes to one, that is worth having,
except as a result of hard work.

— BOOKER T. WASHINGTON

When we asked BLE participants who have lost 100 pounds how they celebrated, some said they haven't because they weren't yet at their goal weight. That seems like a missed opportunity. It is really a diet mentality to wait until we "arrive" to celebrate. We can sabotage ourselves and even slow down our progress. Because in sobriety, there is no "arriving," there is only the next phase of the journey.

We must switch our thinking to realizing that any number of Bright Days accomplished are worth celebrating. However, learning to celebrate without NMF is a skill because our culture relies much too heavily on NMF to signify achievement. And food is always a poor proxy. One woman who achieved a milestone hiked with a friend, took a bubble bath, connected with an old friend, and watched her favorite show. By noting various milestones and learning to celebrate using something other than food, we develop a repertoire of life skills that will keep the journey interesting and enlivened.

ON THIS BRIGHT DAY,

I REFLECT ON WHAT I HAVE ACCOMPLISHED
AND CELEBRATE.

EATING OUT

You can live without anything you weren't born with,
and you can make it through on even half of that.

— GLORIA NAYLOR

Eating out is so doable on BLE. The crux of the issue is how we order when we eat out, because restaurant foods are often made with a lot of oil and butter and what we call "sexier" food ingredients, which can be triggering to the brain. If we are not being honest about eyeballing our portions or using a scale, restaurants can be a pitfall in Maintenance, meaning our choices in restaurants can have a lot to do with whether our weight starts to creep back up and whether our brain gets reactivated into an addictive pattern.

Ultimately, it is worth it to stay vigilant in restaurants to preserve your Bright Transformation and also the peaceful, easy feeling of being able to move freely in the world. By paying attention to how frequently you eat in restaurants and getting curious about your motives (Necessity of your family or work life? A chance to not cook? Entertainment? Indulgence?), you will gain clarity on the role of food in your life—and choose whether you want to continue in that vein.

ON THIS BRIGHT DAY,

I WILL BRING ATTENTION TO MY MOTIVATIONS
BEHIND EATING OUT.

February 19

ENVY

Self-pity in its early stages is as snug as a feather mattress.
Only when it hardens does it become uncomfortable.
— MAYA ANGELOU

Did you spend years being envious of people who are thinner than you? If you lose a lot of weight, are you afraid you will incur the envy of some people dear to you? Envy is an interesting emotion—it lets us know what our heart really desires. Pay attention to what makes you envious and you will have a clue about what you truly want to pursue.

In BLE, we embark on our Bright Transformation in order to pursue our dreams, not as an end in and of itself. Keep your Lines Bright, arrive in your Bright Body, and all along the way listen to what you most want to accomplish, how you most want to spend your time, and what you would like to learn. Use any envy simply as information to act upon, and it will dissipate as you lean into the life you desire.

ON THIS BRIGHT DAY,
I EXPLORE MY FEELINGS OF ENVY FOR CLUES
AS TO WHAT I NEED TO PURSUE.

A LATTICE OF SUPPORT

Your support network is the solid ground from which
you can propel yourself upwards.
— ANNE BARNES

There are so many vehicles of support available on a journey of food sobriety, and we may need every one of them because we live in a hostile food culture where NMF and NMD are normalized and offered, often for free, in so many venues.

When we abstain from sugar and flour and eat only at meals, we are offering our brain the support we need on our journey through life. As we build strong habits in the mornings and evenings, we are providing a structure and scaffolding to help our day be grounded and productive. Having support throughout our day, through multiple media and at different levels of intimacy, can help us navigate challenging situations.

Many of us did not get enough support when we were little, did not know how to ask for it, and used food as our primary coping mechanism. Now we seek human connections, support from pets, the natural world, and a loving and benevolent universe. We also come to appreciate the support we give ourselves.

Learning to lean into this external *and* internal lattice of support is one of the most important skills we develop to soar.

ON THIS BRIGHT DAY,

I LEAN INTO ALL THE FORMS OF SUPPORT ON OFFER AND
EAGERLY PROVIDE SUPPORT TO OTHERS IN TURN.

February 21
COMPLACENCY

It is life near the bone where it is sweetest.
— HENRY DAVID THOREAU

For those further along the BLE path, complacency can be the gateway to a slip. Complacency doesn't always look like not doing what is necessary. Sometimes it looks like externally going through the motions, checking all the boxes, while internally knowing that we are "phoning it in." The challenge is that by the time we realize that doesn't work, we have baked some really bad habits into our program.

If you are not feeling enlivened by the habits that you have developed, you might want to mix up whom you talk with, offer your service to someone who is struggling, or try out a new meditation or movement practice. Keeping the BLE life interesting will make it more sustainable, and getting curious about any complacency is a great place to start.

ON THIS BRIGHT DAY,

I WILL REVISIT THE COMPONENTS OF MY PROGRAM
AND SEE THEM ANEW.

ENGAGE WITH LIFE

Twenty years from now you will be more disappointed by
the things you didn't do than by the ones you did do.
— H. JACKSON BROWN JR.

Having a solid foundation with automaticity and a strong support system is so important because it allows us to engage fully with all of life without worrying first and foremost about food. In the early days of our food sobriety, we may stay away from some social gatherings or events because we worry that we won't be able to navigate the food comfortably. Or we confine ourselves to going out under controlled conditions to a restaurant that we have researched carefully in advance, eating a meal we have committed to a Buddy ahead of time. But while creating a buffer around challenging situations may work initially, eventually we need to engage with all of life. Gradually, we will have built the foundation where we can play a day by ear, be spontaneous with a loved one, and walk into a restaurant we have never been in before and navigate the menu just fine.

Keep in mind that every step you take in the early stages of BLE supports you in having a bold and beautiful life in the world, in the fullness of time.

ON THIS BRIGHT DAY,

I SAY YES TO AN INVITATION I MIGHT HAVE REFUSED.

February 23
SOLITUDE

*The more powerful and original a mind, the more it will
incline towards the religion of solitude.*
— ALDOUS HUXLEY

Many of us ate NMF whenever we found ourselves alone. It was as if being alone was too much without the company of our favorite foods or without the distraction of mindless eating. With the space between three meals each day now looming before us, we have a new opportunity to get acquainted with the peace inherent in solitude. Instead of grazing, what else might we want to do in our precious alone time? How do we make that time replenishing?

What are new practices you may want to cultivate, especially as movement becomes liberated? Yoga? Gardening? Or even reading a book or watching a really great program? Alone time can be a beautiful opportunity for reflection and prayer. Gradually, now that we are Bright, we find ourselves savoring the serenity and peace in our solitude.

ON THIS BRIGHT DAY,
I SEEK A MOMENT OF SOLITUDE AND
NOTICE MY RESPONSE.

February 24
STOP FIGHTING

There is no agony like bearing an untold story inside you.
— ZORA NEALE HURSTON

Anyone who has ever eaten addictively will recognize the feeling of being at war with ourselves. But actually, it is a war between two inner parts of ourselves: the Food Controller and the Food Indulger. They each have their story, and the war between those two can sometimes drive us to insanity. The debate, the struggle, the internal back and forth saps our energy and depletes our willpower.

Did you ever just eat to end the debate? The way to end the war without eating is to hear the stories of the two sides. What does the Indulger need to hear to feel safe? What does the Controller need to hear to feel safe? Hear them both out without judgment and then see how you can make Bright choices that meet their needs. Curiosity is the answer. It ends the battle and gives you peace of mind.

ON THIS BRIGHT DAY,
I CEASE FIGHTING AND LISTEN TO THE INNER PARTS
OF ME THAT NEED TO BE HEARD.

OPENHEARTED

I feel that the human mind has not achieved
anything greater than the ability to share feelings
and thoughts through language.

— JAMES EARL JONES

BLE invites us to open our hearts to others, even when they make mistakes or hurt our feelings. One of the ways to keep our heart open, even to someone who is challenging, is to remember that they, like us, are flawed and human. Approaching things and others openheartedly means feeling the whole spectrum of human emotion, which is actually one of the best parts of being alive.

Without food to modulate emotion, heightening good feelings or numbing what we think of as negative ones, we have an opportunity to step fully into the human experience and trust that our hearts will not only survive but thrive in such an experience. At the same time, being openhearted does not mean giving everything away all the time. Keeping healthy boundaries with our time and our energy can be a vehicle that counterintuitively allows us to be truly openhearted. There is wisdom in asking ourselves, how can we take care of ourselves *and* also show up?

ON THIS BRIGHT DAY,

I WILL WALK THROUGH THE WORLD WITH MY HEART OPEN
AND NOTICE HOW THAT AFFECTS ME AND OTHERS.

February 26
DRIFTING AWAY

Surviving meant being born over and over.
— ERICA JONG

Very few people make a conscious decision to leave this healthy life. Instead, what gradually happens is that without a daily commitment, our anchor habits that keep our Lines Bright erode, the relationships with other Bright Lifers take a back seat to pressing issues, and we suddenly find ourselves on the outside looking in. At that point it is easy to stop making an effort, to pick up the NMF on the way home, and to think we will get started again—tomorrow.

If you find yourself drifting away from the people and the practices that helped you lose your weight and keep your Lines, take notice. It is always possible to turn back toward BLE and your own health and well-being. But just as a few people may decide to leave, those who *decide* to stay have a greater success rate than those who simply hope it will happen. So if you feel yourself drifting away, see what you can do today to reignite your commitment. All of that is in your control.

ON THIS BRIGHT DAY,

I RECOMMIT TO THE BLE PROGRAM AND
BEGIN AS IF THIS IS DAY ONE.

CAPACITY TO LOVE

---

*Love takes off masks that we fear we cannot live without
and know we cannot live within.*

— JAMES BALDWIN

Most of us have a much greater capacity to love than we have evinced through a lifetime of eating NMF, eating round the clock, numbing ourselves with excess food, carrying excess weight, and managing the accompanying health problems. Eating NMF is not self-love and, in many instances, is not loving to others either.

To enhance our capacity to love, we have to uncouple love from food and explore more nuanced and varied options of expression, connection, and intimacy. For example, we can offer to help decorate for a party instead of bringing NMF, or we can bring the new neighbors a potted plant or a beautiful bouquet of flowers instead of NMF. Sometimes simply listening can be one of the greatest acts of love we can perform for someone.

As we recover from our food addiction, we release our self-criticism, doubts, and insecurities—the things that block us from connection. Staying Bright and clear increases our capacity to love and our ability to show up in the present moment. Consider this a new chapter in what your own heart is capable of as you grow in love, courage, kindness, and happiness.

ON THIS BRIGHT DAY,

I LIVE AS IF I HAVE MORE THAN ENOUGH LOVE TO SHARE.

February 28
FORGIVENESS

When you choose not to forgive, the experience
that you do not forgive sticks with you.
— GARY ZUKAV

Hopefully, each of us has at least one someone who has been supportive of us through all kinds of situations. These people are the ones who have known us at our worst and love us anyway. They are special because they have kept a vision of who we truly are and who we can become at the forefront, rather than nursing a long list of our misdeeds.

Conversely, we may hold on to a grudge from our past and keep someone away from our heart, remembering the worst they did to us. But that kind of unforgiveness doesn't harm the other as much as it weighs us down and prevents us from being our best selves.

To forgive, we need to rewrite our grievance story as a story of rising above. Then we need to tell that forgiveness story to ourselves just like we used to repeat the grievance story to ourselves. Through this process we release our resentment and ill will. As we lighten our physical load, we lighten our emotional load and emerge free.

ON THIS BRIGHT DAY,
I WILL SEE WHAT STORIES I CAN REWRITE
WITH COMPASSION AND GRACE.

February 29
IS IT WORKING?

Research is formalized curiosity.
It is poking and prying with a purpose.
— ZORA NEALE HURSTON

Are your Lines Bright? If so, then your program is working. If not, then it is time to level up what you are doing—use more tools and get more support. Shifting something requires leaning into a deeper level of support, upping your inner commitment, and taking more actions that support your Bright Lines.

If you are uncertain what to do differently, talk with someone who is successfully keeping their Lines. Ask how they spend their day—in detail. Chances are high that they are more involved in the BLE program: more faithfully executing their morning and evening habit stacks, more committed to keeping their Lines Bright, making more phone calls, offering more service, and participating more fully in leadership roles than you may be doing currently. Or they may be doing more self-care, taking more walks or naps, or doing more food prep on weekends.

If your own program is not working, apprentice yourself to someone who is feeling more successful and get a blueprint for success to follow.

ON THIS BRIGHT DAY,

I WILL LOOK AT THE RESULTS OF MY BLE PROGRAM
WITH THE EYES OF A RESEARCHER.

March

March 1

PECS

The truth of the matter is, we always know the
right thing to do. The hard part is doing it.
— NORMAN SCHWARZKOPF

Sometimes after a big event like a holiday, a family outing, or the anniversary of a challenging time—something we used to celebrate or survive with NMF—Post-Event Collapse Syndrome (PECS) can occur. Even if we have gotten through the anticipated challenge unscathed, often we let our guard down, and that is when our inner Saboteur or Food Indulger tells us that we deserve a bit more food, a taste of NMF, or a splurge of some kind because we have worked so hard. This can rapidly lead to breaks in our Lines and a time in the ditch, as we say.

Staving off PECS requires planning. Have canned or frozen food available when you return from vacation, so you have meals to tide you over until you can get to the grocery store. Have extra support built into those days after a challenging event and ask your friends to call or text you so you do not have to use energy to reach out. With mindfulness that the times after a significant experience require some forethought and extra gentleness, our growing skill with staying Bright through the whole life cycle of ups and downs becomes a source of pride.

ON THIS BRIGHT DAY,

I WILL LOOK TO THE FUTURE AND SET UP EXTRA
SUPPORT FOR AFTER A BIG EVENT.

PHONE CALLS

What would happen if one woman told the truth
about her life? The world would split open.

— MURIEL RUKEYSER

Everyone in recovery needs support for new habits and behaviors and, while electronic support via online communities, texts, or various apps may be useful, nothing quite buoys us up like face-to-face or voice-to-voice connection. Having real-time connection that picks up every nuance, including silences, emotion, and a quavering voice, works to increase the authentic connection we need in ongoing recovery. This might be why when we have offered programs with rigorous phone call requirements, participants report the greatest change in overall quality of life afterward.

Unfortunately, this easily accessed method can feel very difficult for those of us who have a strong inner Isolator part. Learning to use the phone during easy days serves us during difficult times, because talking on the phone is one of the best ways to get our nervous system to come back into balance when we are in a heightened state of emergency around serious food cravings. Form a group you call regularly who knows the contours of your life and make a schedule to talk regularly. You are weaving a net of support with every single call.

ON THIS BRIGHT DAY,

I WILL CALL SOMEONE AND TELL THEM MY TRUTH.

March 3

ONE DAY AT A TIME

I live a day at a time.
Each day I look for a kernel of excitement.
In the morning, I say:
"What is my exciting thing for today?"
Then, I do the day.
Don't ask me about tomorrow.
— BARBARA C. JORDAN

The word *forever* is often the first line of defense in a food addict's mind. *I cannot possibly do this forever. So maybe I shouldn't even bother . . .*

But we can do *anything* voluntary for 24 hours. And if we can stay sober from sugar and flour for one day, we actually *can* do it for a lifetime. "One day at a time" is a mantra that serves to keep our attention in the now, in today, and works for anything we are trying to do differently. Nobody can imagine living forever without something we have come to depend on. But how about simply getting through the next 24 hours without it? That is doable.

Keeping the focus on the next 24 hours shoos sabotaging brain chatter away and is not a game or a lie, because truly, we all only have this moment, and then the next moment, and then the next. Staying sober one day at a time, one meal at a time, means simply giving this next moment your all. ODAAT is the only path to take.

ON THIS BRIGHT DAY,
I WILL COMMIT FULLY, JUST FOR TODAY.

ACCOUNTABILITY REQUIRES AUTHORITY

If we would have new knowledge,
we must get a whole world of new questions.

— SUSANNE K. LANGER

If we notice our Lines slipping, one of the first things to look at is whether we have imbued our accountability structure with enough authority. If we commit our food on a message board with hundreds of other people, it may not feel binding.

Try setting up a regular (ideally daily) call with someone walking this path. When we connect with them, we will likely be asked some questions: *Did you have a Bright Day yesterday? Have you written down your food? Meditated? Talked to another BLE support person? What are you feeling grateful for today? What are you celebrating?*

Knowing you are going to have to tell the truth to someone tomorrow can often be enough incentive to stick with your food plan today. If you find that you are breaking your Lines, then experiment with different people and systems of reporting until you find the one you care about and respect enough to want to honor through your commitment.

ON THIS BRIGHT DAY,

I WILL FIND THE PERSON I WANT TO UPHOLD
MY INTEGRITY FOR.

FOOD PREPARATION

You do not rise to the level of your goals.
You fall to the level of your systems.
— JAMES CLEAR

Those who keep their Lines Bright under all conditions know that when life gets intense, their food needs to be dialed in even more than usual. The busier your life, the more your food needs to be kept simple and prepared in advance. Setting aside a day each week to do this for the upcoming week is a gift of Brightness you give your future self. It can be a lifesaver as well as a time-saver.

Consider thinking of your food prep as a meditative act of self-care. Chopping vegetables, especially to music or podcasts or other types of nourishing material, can be really calming and relaxing. It can also be a really good time to catch up on a recovery phone call. When it comes to what to prepare, roasting a batch of vegetables, weighing veggies for salads, making rice or oatmeal, or cutting up raw veggies for meals throughout the week helps make BLE meals simple and swift. And when you cook, don't just make one serving of protein or vegetables; make three or four and refrigerate or freeze the rest. You can even weigh out and freeze whole meals to have for later. Leftovers and preparation are a loving gift to your future self.

ON THIS BRIGHT DAY,

I PLAN IN ADVANCE TO SET MYSELF UP FOR SUCCESS.

MARGINS

I never found the companion that was
so companionable as solitude.
— HENRY DAVID THOREAU

When we were eating addictively, many of us were often fueling ourselves with caffeine and sugar and adrenaline to overpower the constant insulin crashes. Even now that we have put down the food, we can still find ourselves addicted to chaos for the adrenaline. It is addictive, and it often takes a lot of recovery to settle into a more peaceful mode of traveling. In addition, many of us ate to signal a transition. We knew intuitively we needed to take a breath and switch gears, but rather than doing just that, we ate something to detach from what we just did and rest before turning to what was next.

Margins of time around activities allow breathing space to transition from one event or person to the next. Making sure you have sufficient time between appointments can eliminate the trigger for food, reduce stress, and make moving into your next appointment a more joyful action. Because we need white space. We write notes in the margins. We pull over on the shoulder of the freeway. And we need to keep margins around our activities because we might need that time—to rest, to recuperate, to transition.

ON THIS BRIGHT DAY,
I MAKE SURE I HAVE ENOUGH TIME FOR ME.

THE THREE Gs

Spiritual empowerment is evidenced in our lives by our
willingness to tell ourselves the truth, to listen to the truth when
it's told to us, and to dispense truth as lovingly as possible,
when we feel compelled to talk from the heart.

— CHRISTINA BALDWIN

There are three Gs on the pathway to achieving surrender:
grace, grit, and gruesomeness.

Grace is when surrender just seems to arrive naturally and
freely—although perhaps not easily or free of pain. We start
Bright Line Eating and we are just willing to do it completely. If
we are on our second, third, or perhaps fortieth go-around, and
we are finding it really hard to stick to the plan, surrender that
emerges from grit is when we force ourselves to just do it one
day at a time. Gruesomeness is when we bang our skull against a
brick wall until we finally just cannot stand the pain anymore—
and a deep shift is borne of utter desperation.

The freedom of surrender is powerful. And often it comes
when we are just too tired to pick up the food one more time.
Surrender requires trust, because we can't always intellectually
understand why something works despite all the wonderful science to support it. Still, trusting that your food is enough, trusting that what has worked for thousands can work for you, and
learning to trust yourself to do the next right thing is the path
to surrender.

ON THIS BRIGHT DAY,

I WILL BECOME MORE WILLING TO SURRENDER TO THE PLAN.

HABIT STACKS

Every action you take is a vote for the type of person you wish to become. No single instance will transform your beliefs, but as the votes build up, so does the evidence of your new identity.

— JAMES CLEAR

Once you commit to following Bright Line Eating, you begin to establish a set of habits that will support this way of eating until it becomes as automatic as brushing your teeth, requiring minimal effort and minimal willpower. Writing down your food the night before becomes reflexive. Weighing out your breakfast in the morning is instinctive. Once you have a habit established, you can add another to it, so that one action leads into the next, with the ending of one behavior cueing the next. This is called a habit stack.

For it truly to be a habit stack, you have to do the actions in the same order, at the same time of day, in the same way. You already do this in all kinds of areas that do not require conscious thought, such as all the micro-tasks involved in showering or driving or making coffee. In BLE, we set in motion habits that nourish our bodies and replenish our willpower, such as meditation, journaling, turning off screens, getting enough sleep, and being of service. And because we have been intentional in setting up good, Bright habits, we are now the recipients of a gift that keeps on giving us the daily scaffolding of a joyous Bright Life.

ON THIS BRIGHT DAY,

I WILL COMPLETE THE SIMPLE TASKS THAT KEEP
MY BLE HABITS STRONG.

NIGHTLY CHECKLIST

What we measure, we improve.

— JAMES CLEAR

Habits you are trying to establish to support a BLE life get reinforced if they are monitored. The easiest way to monitor whether or not you have completed those actions daily is a nightly reflection. Making it a checklist simplifies the time required to review your day and see if you have taken the actions that actually lead to a healed brain.

What is measured and monitored is what is valued, so put on your Nightly Checklist (see Resources on page 383) all the actions you want to be doing. These are actions that nourish you and keep your Lines sparkly Bright, and they may include writing down and committing your food, meditating and moving, talking to supportive BLE people, and anything else you would like to make more automatic in your daily routines. As an action becomes automatic, allow it to fall off the checklist to make space for a new area of growth you want to commit to.

This habit of checking in with yourself and monitoring your progress is a wonderful way to collect data on your journey and see where you may need to adjust the dials on your metaphorical control panel. For example, if you haven't made a support call in a few days, examine that more closely and adjust accordingly. It is your list, so use it to monitor the aspects of your program dearest to you.

ON THIS BRIGHT DAY,

I WILL TRACK THE ACTIONS THAT SUPPORT MY BLE PROGRAM.

SEEK THE LESSON

Every sorrow suggests a thousand songs,
and every song recalls a thousand sorrows, and so
they are infinite in number, and all the same.
— MARILYNNE ROBINSON

While we applaud all our Crystal Vasers—those who have not broken their Bright Lines since getting sober from sugar and flour—we also know that many of us break our Lines and then need to Rezoom. There is never any judgment or shame around someone who has a break, but we urge everyone, every time, to seek the lesson. That requires curiosity and compassion to explore what led up to the break, what the experience was like, and what could be done differently moving forward.

Notice especially if you had warnings or red flags that you ignored. What would have allowed you to heed them instead? That is a fulcrum of opportunity for a major change. Let every break of the Lines lead to greater awareness and a new use of the BLE tools. After all, that is how we grow.

ON THIS BRIGHT DAY,
I WELCOME THE LESSON FROM MY DIFFICULTIES.

March 11

NO EXCEPTIONS,
JUST FOR TODAY

We must disabuse our people of the idea
that there is a shortcut to achievement.
Life requires thorough preparation.
— GEORGE WASHINGTON CARVER

Not making an exception to the plan is the path to success, but most of us cannot conceive of doing *anything* forever, let alone this new way of eating. So adding "just for today" to the "no exceptions" mantra breaks the lifelong goal into small, manageable units.

When your inner Food Indulger suggests that you could have a little NMF and it wouldn't hurt, firmly let it know "no exceptions, just for today." Every break begins with an exception, so if you can keep a firm Line around that, you will never end up in the ditch. Also remember that when it comes to recovery, none is easier than some. The gift of following a no-exceptions policy is a brain that stops suggesting that we deviate, and that is when real peace comes.

ON THIS BRIGHT DAY,

I WILL FOLLOW MY FOOD PLAN WITH
NO EXCEPTIONS—JUST FOR TODAY.

DO NOT SELL YOURSELF SHORT

There is a vitality, a life-force, an energy, a quickening that is translated through you into action and because there is only one of you in all of time, this expression is unique. And if you block it, it will never exist through any other medium and it will be lost.

— MARTHA GRAHAM

Whether it is reaching our goal weight, doing whatever it takes to keep our Lines Bright, or excelling in some area of life completely unrelated to food, many of us stop short of what we truly desire. Maybe we are afraid there will be nothing left to strive for if we get to where we want to go, maybe we carry a sense of unworthiness, or maybe we have never had a champion cheering us on.

Well, in BLE, we are here for you, we know you can get there, and we want you to land in the body and life you truly desire—not one just close enough or almost there. Not one that was within your grasp but got sabotaged by finish-line anxiety. Here is what we know to be true: real peace from food chatter is possible. Real vitality and self-love and buoyancy of spirit are possible. And when we have experienced it in Bright Line Eating, we realize that there is no other way to live.

Keeping your food just sexy enough to keep the food obsession alive is really selling yourself short. Do not compromise on your vision.

ON THIS BRIGHT DAY,

I WILL BELIEVE I CAN HAVE WHAT I TRULY DESIRE.

FLEXIBLE OR BRITTLE FRAMEWORKS

Perfectionism is not the same thing as striving to be our best.
— BRENÉ BROWN

Brittle frameworks come from absolutist, all-or-nothing thinking and counterintuitively disincentivize a return to our goal if we have lapsed even a tiny bit. For example, if you set a New Year's resolution to meditate every single day but miss a couple of days, in a brittle framework you might stop altogether because now there is no way to achieve your goal. You have a flexible framework when you resolve to meditate an average of six days out of seven, so if you miss a couple of days you are incentivized to get right back on track. The goal is not perfection but rather the benefits of the practice itself.

Yet you always want to get back to it as soon as you can. If you break your streak of making support calls, start again as soon as possible. If you miss a few days of exercise, don't beat yourself up—just resume at the next possible opportunity. Because each engagement with that behavior is beneficial. Perfectionism never is. Embrace a flexible framework and you are sure to succeed.

ON THIS BRIGHT DAY,

I WILL NOTICE WHERE I AM INVITED TO BE FLEXIBLE,
WHERE I AM LOOKING TO CUT CORNERS, AND
WHERE I AM HOLDING ON TOO TIGHTLY.

VULNERABILITY

When we were children, we used to think that when we were grown up, we would no longer be vulnerable. But to grow up is to accept vulnerability. . . . To be alive is to be vulnerable.

— MADELEINE L'ENGLE

A happy life is driven by meaningful connection with others. The key to unlocking that connection is vulnerability. It can be very uncomfortable. Often an Isolator part of us is believing a story that if we share our weakness or what is really hard in our lives, others will think less of us. But in truth, it is just the opposite.

Authentic vulnerability requires bravery. Vulnerability means telling the truth, allowing ourselves to feel everything we are feeling, and sharing that with another. Or even ourselves. Every person who begins BLE starts by being vulnerable, acknowledging that what they have been doing has not worked and that they are willing to trust a program, a community of people, and something deep within themselves in order to change.

If you are someone who struggles with perfectionism, allowing yourself to acknowledge the wholeness and fullness of who you are may be the first step in the bravery of being vulnerable with others.

ON THIS BRIGHT DAY,

I WILL LEAN INTO THE VULNERABLE MOMENTS AND
BE TENDER WITH OTHERS DURING THEIRS.

March 15

DEEP COMMITMENT

If one cannot risk oneself, then one is simply incapable of giving.
— JAMES BALDWIN

Deep commitment is what creates the core identity of a Bright Line Eater. But you do not have to be 100 percent committed to BLE every single day; that may not even be humanly possible. The *deeper* your commitment, however, the easier the program becomes.

Some of us have struggled enough before we got into food recovery that we have a powerful drive not to live like we used to, and that alone keeps us deeply committed. For others, deep commitment is built through watching ourselves do the actions. We see ourselves wrangle with our food plan but stick with it, until we have our food for tomorrow written out or abstain from eating NMF at an event when everyone around us seems to be doing nothing but eating, or reach out to make a connection in the community when we feel scared and resistant, and those actions signify our deep commitment. The commitment drives the actions, but then the actions create our lived, felt sense of deep commitment.

And on the days when we do not feel deeply committed, we can keep the commitment alive by doing the actions. Having a deep commitment to not use food to solve a problem means being open and willing to look for solutions elsewhere than we may ever have before. That is how commitment expands our horizons and enlarges our world.

ON THIS BRIGHT DAY,

I COMMIT THROUGH MY ACTIONS.

FOOD OBSESSION

---

*Whatever you give your attention to
is the thing that governs your life.*
— EMMET FOX

Food addiction has a physical *and* a mental component. When you get sugar and flour out of your body, the substances that fan the flames of craving, your brain starts to heal and those pathways become less active, to the point of dormancy. But because addiction abides in the brain *and* the mind, the mental obsession that accompanies the physical addiction lasts longer. Said another way, the physical component of food addiction often means that once we start eating again, we cannot stop. And the mental component means that once we do stop, it is hard to stay stopped.

That is why we have to be vigilant about protecting our mental state and using all the tools of the program. Do not let a dragonfly become a dragon by feeding your random food thoughts. Do not gaze at food, read about it, or entertain thoughts of what it might taste like. Guard the eyes, guard the taste, guard the mind, and turn your attention and energy to what you *do* want.

ON THIS BRIGHT DAY,

I WILL CONSCIOUSLY CHOOSE THOUGHTS THAT BRING
FREEDOM, HAPPINESS, AND LOVE INTO MY WORLD.

USING THE SCALE IN RESTAURANTS

Man is a tool-using animal. . . .
Without tools he is nothing, with tools he is all.
— THOMAS CARLYLE

In order to have our food recovery be really livable, we are going to need to be able to move freely through the world, socialize, and yes, eat out. While keeping our Lines Bright in restaurants is more challenging than at home, the more honest we are and the more tools we use to keep our recovery strong, the more freedom we will find to eat out with peace and ease.

Consider bringing a food scale to restaurants to be assured of success and peace of mind. Asking for an extra plate and then discretely moving the food onto it in exact amounts doesn't require much work and can bring tremendous freedom. If you would rather, simply follow the one-plate rule and eyeball your portions with honest intentions. Ask early for a take-home box and put the extras in it before you eat—that way you aren't tempted to nibble while others finish.

The point of using these tools is so that our minds can be attentive to what truly matters: enjoying the company of others and the ambiance of our dining environment and then walking out of the restaurant mentally free and not second-guessing ourselves or feeling excessively full. Vigilance equals freedom.

ON THIS BRIGHT DAY,

I WILL USE EVERY TOOL AVAILABLE TO KEEP MY LINES BRIGHT IN CHALLENGING SITUATIONS.

March 18

SAYING NO, THANK YOU

Most of us have very weak and flaccid "no" muscles. . . .
Your "no" muscle has to be built up to get to a place where you
can say, "I don't care if that's what you want. I don't want that. No."

— IYANLA VANZANT

Saying, "No, thank you," to someone's offer of NMF should not be complicated or difficult, but the truth is that learning to say it consistently and firmly takes practice. Once we are able to decline any offer without explaining or apologizing, our "no" goes beyond debate or even conversation.

Sometimes when a friend or loved one has worked hard to cook or bake something for us, it feels as if we are not only rejecting their food, we are rejecting them. But that is just a feeling. Food is not love; it is just food. Real love is supporting us in our Bright Journey. If you are heading into a challenging situation in which you may have to say, "No, thank you," repeatedly, spend time reviewing all the reasons you work this program and everything you will get to say yes to as a result. It is much easier to say a firm, "No, thank you," when you have a clear sense of what you are saying yes to instead: clarity of mind, a Bright Body, freedom from compulsions, and true integrity.

ON THIS BRIGHT DAY,

I WILL SPEAK HONESTLY AND KNOW I DO NOT
EVER OWE ANYONE A BITE OF NMF.

SADNESS

> If we had no winter, the spring would not be so pleasant:
> if we did not sometimes taste of adversity,
> prosperity would not be so welcome.
> — ANNE BRADSTREET

Sadness is part of the human experience, yet so many of us used to avoid it, or thought we did, by eating something to distract or soothe us. It is true that NMF provides a hit of dopamine and lifts us above a temporary state of boredom or despair, but repeated ingestion of NMF dulls the spectrum of human emotion to the point where we need a hit of NMF to even feel normal.

Periodic feelings of sadness are a healthy part of life. Learning to ride that wave of feeling—to be present, curious, and compassionate to what is going on within us—not only allows us to move through life without the crutch of food, it expands our capacity to be present and of service to others who are experiencing difficult emotions.

If we use the tool BFF—Breathe, Feel your body, Find your feet (or your seat)—we can tune into the feeling in our body and sit with it mindfully. By just breathing in and out without judgment or any urgency or agenda, we will find that every feeling, no matter what feeling it is, will pass. If each time we feel a feeling, we just tune into the physical sensation of it, we can become quite skilled at riding the ebb and flow of being deliciously alive.

ON THIS BRIGHT DAY,
I STOP, BREATHE, AND WELCOME ALL THAT I AM FEELING.

March 20

SELF-SUPPORT

If we intend merely to coast along the low roads,
maybe we can do it alone. If we are heading for the mountains,
the support of others is indispensable.

— MICHAEL CASEY

There is a fine line between relying on oneself, going deep within to find the strength to do hard things, and the overreliance on self where we spurn others' help. It is true that we need to make the inner decision to live the BLE way of life, and yet we cannot do it alone. Conversely, while we need a community of support to get through hard things, nobody can actually do this program for us. How do we know where the line is between sufficient self-support and overreliance?

One question we can ask ourselves is: *How deeply supported and connected am I feeling on my Bright Journey right now?* There can be an awful lot of autonomous, self-directed, and productive activity within a container of feeling deeply supported and connected. But if we feel like we are dangling out there alone—if we feel lonely or isolated—then when adversity strikes, we are not going to have the resources to overcome it. We can pay attention to how we feel, notice what being out-of-balance feels like, and make a small adjustment by calling someone, asking for help, or offering our listening ear to someone in pain.

ON THIS BRIGHT DAY,

I WILL SUPPORT BOTH MYSELF AND OTHERS
AND SEEK THE SAME.

EMBRACING ENOUGH

If [enough] was really something out there—
a definable quantity—then everyone who had that
quantity would know they had enough.

— GENEEN ROTH

Those of us who are inclined toward addiction, who crave do-pamine, the molecule of more, tend to run to extremes and do not necessarily have the natural magnetism toward modera-tion that others have. Those of us who habitually ate too much food may not have any idea what "enough" is, so we rely on the BLE food plan to provide our bodies the right amount of food to thrive and lose weight. That intuitive sense of what is enough food may never be restored in us, and that's okay, because we can always rely on the scale to tell us proper portions.

Paying attention to what is enough in other areas of life—like clothes, affection, attention, movement, wealth, tidiness, or work—can be an adventure. If we stay dopamine dominant, we're going to always be striving. So we nurture the serotonin, oxytocin, and endorphins in our brains, the here-and-now mole-cules, so we won't need as much striving in our lives to feel good. That means sometimes the feeling of having or being enough is just a brisk walk or a big hug away.

ON THIS BRIGHT DAY,
I WILL TUNE INTO WHAT ENOUGH FEELS LIKE.

YES AND NO

---

*The oldest, shortest words—yes and no—
are those which require the most thought.*

— PYTHAGORAS

It can be very hard for some of us to say no. We do not want to let people down, make them mad, or hurt their feelings. Even worse, we do not want to ruin a relationship. Except that when we are not honest with others, or ourselves, when we caretake and placate and are codependent by saying yes when we really should be saying no, we start to erode the integrity of our relationships. But even more, when we say yes when we want to say no, we set ourselves up for resentment and can end up looking for compensation, which often takes the form of food.

We learn over time that every yes involves a lot of nos. When we say yes to a vacation, it means disrupting our solid routines back home. When we say yes to a move, it means leaving friends behind. Being open to one experience or adventure necessitates turning away from others. Conversely, when we say no to NMF and NMD, we are saying yes to our best and Brightest selves. Learning to embrace *no* is a powerful part of this journey.

ON THIS BRIGHT DAY,
I WILL HONOR THE "NO" IN ME AND EXPRESS IT.

March 23

SURRENDER

Surrender to what *is*. Say "yes" to life—and see how life starts suddenly starts working *for* you rather than against you.

— ECKHART TOLLE

Surrender—the willingness to do whatever it takes to follow our plan just for today—is the foundation of working a program of food recovery. It is the moment we wave the white flag and accept that we just cannot do this by ourselves, admitting that all the things we have been doing to try to manage our food have not been working.

There is a powerful feeling when you surrender, and it is often as emotional as it is physical. For many of us, it is spurred by hitting a number on the scale that we never thought we would hit, or going on a binge that renders us practically unable to move or breathe without pain, or getting a health diagnosis that scares us straight. You might want to think of surrender as a switch you flip on once to have all the light you need. But most of us experience it as a dimmer switch that can always grow brighter and never goes out completely. In other words, any time you come face-to-face with resistance to follow the BLE plan, you have an opportunity to surrender yet again.

ON THIS BRIGHT DAY,

I EMBRACE SURRENDERING TO THE PLAN.

END THE DEBATE

> To win, or to create a great group with winning mentality,
> you need first stability, but serenity as well. And it is only by
> creating an internal and mutual trust that you can achieve it.
>
> — MATTIA BINOTTO

The debate between our inner Food Indulger and Food Controller was exhausting, and most of us ended the debate by capitulating, knowing full well we would eventually—so why not get it over with? The new way to end the debate in BLE is to not let it even begin.

Every morning we wake up and commit to following the plan, to doing whatever it takes to not pick up food as a means to cope with life. The gift of BLE is the serenity in our minds once the decision has been made not to eat sugar or flour, not to snack, and not to overeat—to eat only and exactly what we wrote down the night before. Eventually, that becomes the most familiar path in our brains and automatically enables us to move through the world in a blessed state of food neutrality.

Keeping our Lines Bright will end the debate about whether or not to eat, whether or not to stop eating, and even whether or not to tell someone the truth about our eating. It is a tremendous blessing.

ON THIS BRIGHT DAY,

I QUIET MY MIND AND MOVE TOWARD MY HEART'S DESIRE.

INNER STRENGTH

This inner strength we have, this desire to evolve and
expand and explore, I do love that about humanity.

— MATT BELLAMY

Support from others will make a tremendous difference in the
success of your BLE journey, but everyone who keeps their
Lines Bright also draws upon inner strength and resources, or
what psychologists call grit. Because, as helpful as other people
are, they are not always available, and we have to begin to count
on ourselves to get through some challenging times. Ultimately,
we are the guardians of our minds.

We do not have much control over a first thought, but we
have a lot of control over what happens after that. Every day,
spend some time cultivating that fortitude and strength of mind.
It can be nurtured and reinforced through meditation and the use
of mantras. Each time we go within and reflect, we touch upon
our inner resolve. Activating a reserve of willingness strengthens
your chance to do that again tomorrow.

ON THIS BRIGHT DAY,

I WILL DRAW UPON MY INNER STRENGTH.

March 26
WISDOM

When we are able to value our self-worth as much as we listen to the self-critic, we begin to tap the resource of wisdom.
— ANGELES ARRIEN

When it comes to wisdom in recovery, we want to cultivate it within—and without. Leaning into external wisdom means listening to the experience of thousands who have successfully worked the BLE program before us. We follow the plan, recommendations, and guidance of experienced coaches and successful members.

Our bodies have an innate wisdom that some of us have overridden for years, filling ourselves with food that was not beneficial to our health or eating too much or too restrictively. Because of years of disordered eating, most of us cannot eat intuitively. Our brains are just not wired that way. For this reason, to cultivate our own inner wisdom we must learn to tune into how much support we need, what kind, and which foods within each category we thrive on.

Learning to trust our own wisdom means sometimes ignoring it and noticing the consequences—paying attention to the results—and always being on the lookout for guidance from within and without that resonates with our inner knowing.

ON THIS BRIGHT DAY,
I GATHER THE PEARLS OF WISDOM FROM EVERYONE
AROUND ME AND FROM DEEP INSIDE.

LIMITING BELIEFS

That is what learning is. You suddenly understand something you've understood all your life, but in a new way.

— DORIS LESSING

It is inevitable that many of us will come to BLE with a diet mentality and preconceived ideas about weight loss and what we can and cannot do. Having tried numerous approaches, we have developed a self-concept as someone who simply cannot succeed. Rehearsing arguments in our head, scripting a situation to control the outcome, and worrying rather than preparing for a challenging food situation all stem from old ideas of how we navigate the world. It takes nuanced skill to notice how subtly our old ideas can interfere with or limit today's happiness.

But every day is an invitation to notice and release the ideas that no longer serve us. By starting fresh every day and asking for help when we find ourselves in uncharted territory, our ideas will be refreshed, our spirit will be renewed, and we will find the combination of willingness and tools to create a reality well beyond anything we could have imagined possible.

ON THIS BRIGHT DAY,

I RELEASE ANY IDEA ABOUT MYSELF THAT
NO LONGER SERVES ME.

DAILY DEPOSITS

*With consistency and reps and routine you're going to
achieve your goals and get where you want to be.*
— MANDY ROSE

Working a BLE program one day at a time means we have to do something to contribute to our forward momentum every single day. When we look at someone who has had their Bright Transformation and is flourishing, it might seem like they have something that is out of reach for us. But the reality is that they built that Bright Transformation through a series of small daily actions.

We start off by writing down our food the night before and committing it, and then the next day eating only and exactly that. After we have done that for a few weeks, those daily deposits start to yield interest because we find ourselves in a state where it does not take much energy to continue. Regardless of what we have done in the past, we can start today by making our daily deposits. That may mean professing our identity as a Bright Line Eater out loud to ourselves before we head into the grocery store or picking up the phone, even when we are tired. Acknowledging, affirming, and moving toward our BLE identity is a daily deposit that will pay off when we face the next challenging time.

ON THIS BRIGHT DAY,

I WILL PUT MONEY IN THE BANK TOWARD
MY BRIGHT TRANSFORMATION BY TAKING THE
ACTIONS THAT SUPPORT ME.

March 29
NO DECISIONS

---

*If you think that you are bound, you remain bound;
you make your own bondage. If you know that you are free,
you are free this moment. This is knowledge,
knowledge of freedom. Freedom is the goal of all nature.*

— SWAMI VIVEKANANDA

Let us take today to remember that the anterior singular cortex, the center of decision-making in the brain, gets fatigued through the myriad activities of a hectic modern life. It is trying to help us regulate our emotions and stay on track with complex tasks and resist temptations. When it gets fatigued, we fall into the Willpower Gap.

If we leave our Bright Transformation in the hands of dozens of momentary food-related decisions all throughout the day, we are sunk. Having Bright Lines takes the decision-making out of the hundreds of food choices we are faced with every day, and that means our willpower will not be so depleted that we will fall back on old neural pathways for comfort and ease.

By writing down our food the night before and then making *one* decision in the morning—to stick to our food plan—we now have more mental space and energy for the really important decisions we will face today. We embrace the day with the gift of freedom that our food is dialed in and we do not need to obsess about what, when, and how much to eat today.

ON THIS BRIGHT DAY,

I WILL SIMPLY FOLLOW THE PLAN
AND ENJOY THAT FREEDOM.

START OVER ANYTIME

> You may have a fresh start any moment you choose,
> for this thing that we call "failure" is not the falling down,
> but the staying down.
> — MARY PICKFORD

There is something auspicious about January 1, Monday morning, or 8 A.M. as a time to begin anew. But in BLE, if we slip, we Rezoom, quickly starting over with the next meal or the next moment. By taking the power of beginning into this moment, we create endless possibilities for renewal and do not reinforce the old what-the-hell mentality that said, *I have already messed up—might as well eat everything I have not had for a while and start over tomorrow.* The truth is, every single extra bite of NMF we eat makes it that much harder to return to our program; so we turn back onto the Bright path as fast as possible.

Being unstoppable is what matters most, and that can happen in every moment.

ON THIS BRIGHT DAY,
I GIVE MYSELF PERMISSION TO
START OVER AT ANY POINT.

March 31
INCREMENTAL PROGRESS

We do not remember days, we remember moments.
— CESARE PAVESE

Magical thinking had some of us trying fad diets, taking pills, or starving ourselves for crash weight loss. After all that, at first the steady progress of following BLE can feel too slow for some of us. We are not used to noticing incremental progress, trusting a program to deliver us to our Bright Body if we stick with it. And we are definitely not used to being happy along the way.

Postponing happiness until we reach our goal does not guarantee we will get there. Instead, enjoying every bit of progress we are making and trusting that we will arrive when the time is right will lead to a real shift in our identity and the cultivation of a mindset that makes Maintenance sustainable.

In order to notice week-to-week progress, we have to pay attention to more subtle changes than a number on the scale. Learning to notice a greater freedom of movement, a clarity of mind, or a state of contentment happens with fine-tuned attention. These major gifts of Bright Line Eating get delivered well before we are living in our Bright Body.

ON THIS BRIGHT DAY,

I WILL TRUST THAT MY BRIGHT TRANSFORMATION IS
HAPPENING INCREMENTALLY, RIGHT ON SCHEDULE.

April

April 1

BLTS

Eat food. Not too much. Mostly plants.
— MICHAEL POLLAN

Bites, Licks, and Tastes (BLTs) may seem innocuous—after all, you are going to eat pretty soon and it is BLE-compliant food, right? Of course the issue is not the calories—a morsel of carrot off a cutting board is trivial from a caloric perspective—but the problem of keeping our process addiction alive. The first two Bright Lines, Sugar and Flour, address the substance side of food addiction. And the last two Bright Lines, Meals and Quantities, address the process side.

When we engage in BLTs, we are fostering a brain that constantly asks, *Is it time to eat yet? Can I have a little bit more? How about now? How about now?* That is not peace and that is not freedom. Also, breaking the Line of eating only at meals can provide a toehold for our inner Saboteur to make an exception and then another. By keeping our Lines sparkly Bright, we shore up our identity as someone who never makes an exception, and that heals our brain and serves us best in the long run. After all, a brain that makes exceptions with a bite or taste could also make an exception for NMF when the opportunity presents itself.

ON THIS BRIGHT DAY,

I WILL KEEP MY LINES SPARKLY BRIGHT ALL DAY LONG.

April 2

RECEIVING HELP

There is no need to struggle to be free;
the absence of struggle is in itself freedom.

— CHOGYAM TRUNGPA

A lot of us come to our food journey with a history of being of service to others before doing for ourselves. We are often way more inclined to give help, but learning how to receive is an important skill.

If you are someone who is giving, but has a hard time receiving, try starting by simply receiving wisdom from anyone who has experience on the BLE journey. Open yourself up with a question, with curiosity. Try receiving a compliment with a heartfelt thank-you rather than a deflection. Try seeing people's offers of help as genuine and accept that help. It is an important skill to learn how to raise your hand, ask for help, and accept it. Because isolation is exactly what our inner addict would love for us to experience, nobody can recover from addiction alone.

Allowing yourself to receive help means you are part of a community, you belong, and you are deserving of others' time and attention. When giving and receiving are a fluid, ongoing experience, well-being occurs, and we create a healthy, permeable life.

ON THIS BRIGHT DAY,
I GLADLY RECEIVE THE SUPPORT, CONNECTION,
AND KINDNESS THIS WORLD OFFERS.

April 3
MEDITATION

Meditation is a vital practice to access conscious
contact with your highest self.
— WAYNE DYER

Research shows that consistent meditators experience a shift in prefrontal cortex activity from the right hemisphere to the left, which means a shift from the grumpy, depressive, dissatisfied part of our brain to the grateful, contented, joyful part. Meditation literally produces happiness—in as little as 10 minutes a day! Of course, when we sit in meditation, we can have monkey mind, which in the past may have felt uncomfortable because our expectation may have been to quiet the mind. But today we can come into our meditation practice with a commitment to be curious about where the mind goes.

The effect of a consistent meditation practice is like stepping onto a moving sidewalk in an airport. You are still going from point A to point B, but the journey itself is easier and more enjoyable. The additional boost from meditation comes from healing the brain, tapping into the highest vibrational energy available, and bringing all parts of ourselves into alignment so we are more calm, clear, and connected.

ON THIS BRIGHT DAY,
I WILL SIT IN MEDITATION AND SIMPLY BREATHE.

BOOKENDING

> Lots of people want to ride with you in the limo,
> but what you want is someone who will take the bus
> with you when the limo breaks down.
> — OPRAH WINFREY

Bookending is a practice of accountability. Before you go into a challenging situation or event, let someone in the community know that you intend to keep your Lines Bright. When the event is over, let them know that, in fact, you did stick to your Lines. If you didn't, tell them that too. Knowing that you are going to have to report the truth at the end of the situation is an added incentive to keep to your Lines.

The hardest situations for sticking to our food plan are celebrations held in restaurants, parties, and other special events. But sometimes when we are new on our journey in recovery, just going to the grocery store can be really challenging and a great activity to bookend. An added benefit is that when we let people know we are vulnerable, it builds community. Then later they will be there to remind us once those same events or situations have gotten easier. When we let other people into our journey deeply, we all benefit. Just like bookends hold a stack of books upright, so can your bookend support your Bright Lines.

ON THIS BRIGHT DAY,

I TRUST ANOTHER TO HELP SUPPORT ME AND
CELEBRATE MY VICTORY AS WELL.

SANE CHOICES

You must always be able to predict what's next and
then have the flexibility to evolve.
— MARC BENIOFF

At first, as your brain heals, your inner Indulger will keep wanting you to wriggle out of this new commitment, so rigidly applying BLE principles to every single context possible is the way to go. But as you gain automaticity and begin to identify as a Bright Lifer, you may need to discern what works and what will be workable given a circumstance. Sometimes life gets lifey.

For example, you discover your broccoli got slimy. Don't eat it. But don't abandon your entire plan either. Grab a can or some frozen veggies and make a quick swap. If you want to be really clean about it, commit the change to someone. This is different than making a swap because we want to. The goal is to make that entire seeking-a-hit-from-the-food impulse go extinct in our brain. We want to have a brain that is peaceful, calm, and quiet, and we do that by not encouraging spur-of-the-moment changes.

The question is one of motives: Is my inner Indulger calling the shots or is the sanest part of me suggesting a shift given these circumstances? Over time you will learn to trust yourself to make that distinction.

ON THIS BRIGHT DAY,
I WILL NOTICE MY MOTIVES AND ALIGN
MY ACTIONS ACCORDINGLY.

A BIG ENOUGH WHY

He whose life has a why can bear most any how.
— FRIEDRICH NIETZSCHE

It can be hard to recall with a powerful force the mental state that we were in when we chose to start this journey—how bleakly trapped we felt and how desperate for a solution we were. If we have not had our Bright Transformation yet, it is time to reflect deeply on the question, *Why am I doing this?* When you reach your Bright Body, what will sustain eating this way? Having a reason to eat Bright beyond getting a different pants size is important for creating a new identity.

That is where your "why" comes in. Whether it is for health, happiness, or the freed-up energy available to pursue other passions, getting clear on *why* you want to end this addiction cycle with food can serve you now and going forward. For many it is that we come to feel profoundly differently about ourselves by working this program, and the restored integrity and self-esteem is worth it on every level.

ON THIS BRIGHT DAY,

I WILL REFLECT ON MY "BIG WHY" AND
CELEBRATE THAT I CHOOSE TO BE BRIGHT.

CHILDHOOD STORIES

I'd always been enthralled by stories of wreckage.
But I wanted to know if stories about getting better could
ever be as compelling as stories about falling apart.
I needed to believe they could.

— LESLIE JAMISON

So many of our favorite foods are connected with pleasant memories from our childhood. We tell ourselves a story that life won't be sweet without a certain NMF, that we won't feel part of our family holiday gathering if we don't participate in eating the traditional NMF, or that people will be disappointed if we don't bring the NMF dish everyone loves. What will they think of us?

These stories are, in actuality, childish, because when we think of the reason we connect with family, celebrate holidays, or make occasions special, food does not need to be the center-piece. In fact, food is a poor proxy for connection. Instead, focus on conversation, pitching in outside of the kitchen, and joining in on the activities you may have missed in the past because you were so focused on the food. We can bring a new kind of child-like joy and energy to holidays by keeping our Lines Bright and focusing on the people in the room.

ON THIS BRIGHT DAY,

I WILL SHARE A HAPPY MEMORY WITH SOMEONE I LOVE.

LIVE IN COLOR

Sunset is still my favorite color, and rainbow is second.
— MATTIE STEPANEK

In the throes of addiction, it may have felt like we were living in black and white. As our world shrank to accommodate our bottomless need for NMF, we may have gradually allowed our lives to dim, with the light of human connection and true joy fading away. As our brains became increasingly hijacked, it may have felt like the world had nothing to offer us beyond the next hit. Additionally, think back to how you were eating then. How much of your food was white? White flour, white sugar, white starch, white entrees with white sauce and white sides.

One of the great joys of living Bright is also eating Bright. At every meal we invite the rainbow to our table. Orange and purple carrots, deep green leaves, red seeds, blue berries. This diversity is nutritionally optimal and a delight for the senses.

As we work the program and heal and connect with others and our higher purpose, we now get to live—and eat—in glorious technicolor. See what colors you can taste in your next Bright meal.

ON THIS BRIGHT DAY,
I SAVOR ALL THE NUTRITIOUS FLAVORS
OF NATURE'S RAINBOW.

April 9
WHOLE FOODS

A world without tomatoes is like a
string quartet without violins.
— LAURIE COLWIN

Many of us come into Bright Line Eating with brains so impacted by ultra-processed foods that eating real food can be difficult at first. Research shows that when rats are fed a diet consisting of NMF, they acclimate to it very quickly and gain a ton of weight. When they get put back on basic rat pellets, they will literally starve themselves to death rather than eat those.[1]

Luckily our brain does heal quickly, and over time we come to love the wholesome, real vegetables that we eat in this program. In fact, it becomes a source of never-ending delight. If you are struggling, ask a BLE friend for preparation suggestions or consult the official cookbook, which is devoted to initiating people to the joys of vegetables. Soon you will be able to discern the sweetness of a carrot and the delicious variety across many types of apples, and your eyes will delight in the rich rainbow on your plate. Best of all, you will have the satisfaction of knowing that you are nourishing your mind, body, and spirit with every bite.

ON THIS BRIGHT DAY,
I SAVOR THE AMAZING PRODUCE ON MY PLATE.

YOUR SUPPORT BAR

The greatest weapon against stress is our ability
to choose one thought over another.

— WILLIAM JAMES

Daily life has stress built into it. A stress-free life would be one without family, without work, without connection. Truly, any meaningful connection or pursuit comes with some stress and challenges. But no matter the level of stress in your life, you need to have more support than stress; otherwise, your inner Indulger will wedge itself into that gap.

It is important to assess how much support you have for the current circumstances of your life, and if it is not enough, increase it. How do you assess your level of stress? Give it a rating on a 1–10 scale or make a bar graph you update daily. Give yourself a visual metric of what you are up against right now. Then match that with your support.

Support could be physical rejuvenation, ample sleep, time in nature, or unstructured downtime. It could be increased social support, hugs, or touch connection with people that you love. You might be tempted to cut back on these activities when you're stressed because you feel like you do not have any free time. But that is counterproductive. Raise your support to match your stressors and NMF will never seem like the answer.

ON THIS BRIGHT DAY,

I WILL STRENGTHEN THE SUPPORT I HAVE BY THANKING THOSE
WHO ALREADY SUPPORT ME—AND ASKING FOR MORE.

April 11
THINK LONG TERM

A man who is a master of patience is master of everything else.
— GEORGE SAVILE

We tend to be an impatient lot, not used to delayed gratification nor able to see the long view. Slow but steady weight loss may not feel dramatic enough, and unfortunately, that can lead to discouragement and broken Lines. But know that profound transformations, especially from big numbers, take time.

It took us years to eat ourselves into misery, and it may take more than a few months to eat our way out. In order to move through the weight-loss phase of BLE with ease, you need a big picture. BLE is *not* a diet—it is a lifestyle choice—so it does not make a difference how long it takes. If the scale is not budging as fast as we would like, we might be getting on it too frequently—and it does not serve us to do that.

The main thing to focus on is keeping our Lines Bright just for today. As we do that, the scale will move in the right direction, no matter the pace, and our accepting and positive attitude will keep us beyond NMF temptation. If we focus on our Bright Lines, we will lose the weight. But if we focus on the weight, we will lose our Bright Lines.

ON THIS BRIGHT DAY,
I FOCUS ON THE BIG PICTURE AND
ENJOY THE JOURNEY.

April 12
CUTTING CORNERS

We have to try to cure our faults by attention and not by will.
— SIMONE WEIL

Doing anything precisely the same day after day takes discipline and conscious attention to the process. If we are focused on getting results and not paying attention to how enjoyable and life-giving each task in the day can be, we may be tempted to let up on the thoroughness of our program in order to "arrive."

Cutting corners by jumping up before our meditation timer goes off, for example, or skipping committing our meals is a sign that we are too focused on the outcome and not enough on the process or journey. Playing fast and loose in a seemingly innocuous area may quickly escalate into a break in our Lines, so we look to see where we may need to tighten up. Maybe it is making our support calls or reinstating our morning habit stack or our nightly self-assessment. Maybe we have just started eyeballing all our portions. Whatever it may be, today is a great day to get those corners Bright and sharp again.

ON THIS BRIGHT DAY,
I WILL GIVE MY FULL ATTENTION TO
CRISPING UP MY PROGRAM.

BALANCING SERVICE AND SELF-CARE

*I would find no interest in living in an age
when there were no weak members of the human
family to be helped, no wrongs to be righted.*

— BOOKER T. WASHINGTON

Service can be an important component of this recovery program. Our BLE online support community is filled with people who offer their experience and their encouragement to others freely. But focusing on helping others at the detriment of taking time for yourself can create an imbalance that eventually leads to resentment and perhaps rationalizing the consolation prize of NMF.

Balancing service with self-care means paying attention to our energy levels and noticing if we are giving freely or keeping score and expecting to be thanked. These are indicators that we may not be giving from our Authentic Self and it is time to nurture and replenish ourselves before we perform another act in service of others.

ON THIS BRIGHT DAY,
I NOTICE WHEN I NEED SELF-CARE
AND WHEN I WANT TO HELP.

REACH OUT FIRST

Loneliness is proof that your innate search
for connection is intact.
— MARTHA BECK

Addiction works best in isolation, so notice if you are reluctant to talk to someone before taking a bite off the BLE food plan. Reaching out before taking that bite will not only keep your Lines Bright but also reinforce your identity as someone who knows the answer to any need lies in greater connection, not in consuming something. We want to get to a place in Bright Line Eating where we have people to call when we are feeling in jeopardy of picking up an addictive bite of food off our plan.

It takes time to nurture a circle of support, but it is something that is worth investing in. If we have not been reaching out on happy days, lazy Tuesday afternoons, and everything in between, we will not take that action when we need it most.

ON THIS BRIGHT DAY,

I WILL ASK FOR SUPPORT, KNOWING IT WILL
BENEFIT THE GIVER AS WELL.

April 15
FIND A GUIDE

We grant authority to people we perceive as "authoring"
their own words and actions, people who do not speak from
a script or behave in pre-programmed ways.
— PARKER PALMER

A Guide is someone who offers temporary support to someone who is struggling or in transition. Often we do not need a Guide at first because our program is laid out very simply and cleanly and the materials themselves take our hand and show us how to get started. But if we find ourselves in the ditch or struggling with repeated patterns of breaking our Lines—or we simply want to take our program to a new level—finding someone in the community who embodies the kind of Bright Line Eating program we would like to manifest can be a tremendous support.

A Guide is someone who has immaculate Bright Lines, works a strong program, and has the time to offer support and accountability to someone who requests it. It is a one-way relationship (unlike the one with a Buddy), and you should discuss an end date before it even begins. Transitioning from the support of a Guide to the support of the BLE community is the goal, where once you have reestablished your Bright Lines, you can look ahead to the day when you will become someone else's Guide.

ON THIS BRIGHT DAY,
I WILL EXPLORE WHETHER I NEED EXTRA SUPPORT
TO STRENGTHEN MY PROGRAM.

April 16

BRUSH FOOD THOUGHTS AWAY

The greatest discovery of my generation is that human beings can alter their lives by altering their attitudes of mind.

— WILLIAM JAMES

Everyone thinks about eating off plan from time to time. In the beginning of BLE or after a series of breaks and Rezooms, those thoughts may come quite frequently. This is not a bad sign. Food thoughts are natural. At first, they might be so powerful as to feel overwhelming; but over time, they will become fainter until you hardly notice them. However, the thought is one thing, while nurturing it and feeding it so that it becomes a plan is a whole other animal.

That is why it is important not to feed those thoughts but instead to brush them off with a mantra, like "That's not my food—it's poison to me." Or by turning your attention to something that *is* nourishing, like "I am so grateful for my Buddy and this community." If we feed negative thoughts intermittently by breaking our Lines, they will be profoundly resistant to extinction and plague us for a long, long time. But by brushing away food thoughts, we let our inner Indulger know we will not be going down that path; eventually those thoughts diminish and, for some folks, go away almost entirely. Firmly turning away those thoughts today gives your future self the opportunity for peace.

ON THIS BRIGHT DAY,

I FEED ONLY THOSE THOUGHTS THAT
SERVE MY AUTHENTIC SELF.

ONE-PLATE RULE

Daring to set boundaries is about having the courage to love ourselves, even when we risk disappointing others.

— BRENÉ BROWN

The dance of sobriety is that we commit to restrictions to find freedom from the shackles of addiction. We push ourselves out of our isolated comfort zone to heal while also respecting that not every aspect of the program will work for every person.

For this reason, when it comes to our fourth Bright Line, Quantities, some people choose not to weigh their food on a digital scale but use the one-plate rule, which is exactly as it sounds. All our food fits on one plate and we do not have seconds. This rule can work for those who would rather not bring a scale to a restaurant, a friend's house, or a buffet line. This is not a chance to game the system, however. We do not use the one-plate rule and then pile it high with grains or oily roasted vegetables or twice the protein portion we would normally have. The one-plate rule requires integrity and honest eyeballing of portions.

If your Authentic Self is calling on you to try this, run the experiment. If your weight stays in check and you continue to feel free and calm, then you have added another tool to your sobriety arsenal.

ON THIS BRIGHT DAY,

I PUT A BOUNDARY AROUND MY FOOD
IN ORDER TO HAVE FREEDOM.

RED FLAGS

History is a vast early warning system.
— NORMAN COUSINS

Most people break their Lines after a series of bumps that signaled that their Lines were not as shiny Bright as they could be. Those indicators differ from person to person, so it is crucial that you learn what indicates a slip for you and tighten up as soon as possible.

For some of us, it is eating out in restaurants more often. Others start choosing bigger and bigger fruits or using excessive condiments. Still others' Lines grow wonky when they skip writing down their food for a day or two. Wonky Lines are like the bumps on the side of the highway that indicate that you have crossed out of your lane. The sooner you notice, the smaller the adjustment you will have to make. The longer you ignore the indicators, the more likely you are headed into the ditch. Check your instrument panel and adjust accordingly. If you need to reach out for added support, there is no embarrassment in admitting you have been swerving; we are here for you.

ON THIS BRIGHT DAY,

I PAY CLOSE ATTENTION TO ALL ASPECTS OF MY PROGRAM
AND COURSE-CORRECT AS NEEDED.

April 19
REGRET

Regret for the things we did can be tempered by time;
it is regret for the things we did not do that is inconsolable.
— SYDNEY J. HARRIS

If we have spent a lot of time obsessed with our food and weight, regret is an old frenemy. But we must learn to let go of past regrets. We must know and trust that as we live Bright one day at a time, we will be uniquely qualified to be of service to others. Similarly, we will never regret keeping our Lines Bright, ever. No matter how tempting the NMF, how special the occasion, or how stressful the experience, sticking to our BLE food plan is a foolproof insurance plan against a regret hangover tomorrow.

When tempted, some people are able to think through the situation to its natural conclusion and anticipate the future pain the momentary indulgence will cause. Others work with newcomers or those recently Rezooming to be reminded of the inevitable regret people feel when they break their Lines. Skip the regret and just follow the plan. Because now that you have strengthened the neuropathway for healthy Bright Line Eating, next time the occasion will be less challenging and the NMF less tempting. And that is the opposite of regret—that is sailing through Bright and shiny!

ON THIS BRIGHT DAY,

I WILL RELEASE REGRET FOR THE PAST AND MAKE THE
CHOICE TO AVOID REGRET IN THE FUTURE.

QUESTIONS OPEN THE MIND

A closed mind is a dying mind.
— EDNA FERBER

Curiosity is one of the 8 Cs of the Authentic Self and, coupled with compassion, will supply a tremendous amount of insight on our journey. This is as true with others as it is with ourselves. For example, curiosity and compassion can help elucidate all the reasons that in the past we might have used food to meet needs other than hunger. By maintaining an open, curious, compassionate state, we will see what we need to see when it is time to see it; we will come to trust that we always receive the guidance we need.

When our system is telling us we need to eat, curiosity about what we really need might reveal that we need rest, fun, connection, or celebration. By honestly asking, *What is going on here?* when you have a food thought, temptation, or craving, you invite an answer from your innermost self. Sometimes those answers are quite surprising. It is best to keep an open mind and use questions rather than advice-giving when working with yourself, and others as well.

ON THIS BRIGHT DAY,

I WILL ASK QUESTIONS, FOLLOW MY CURIOSITY,
AND BRING COMPASSION TO MYSELF AND OTHERS.

BEAUTY

To seek after beauty as an end, is a wild goose chase,
a will-o'-the-wisp, because it is to misunderstand
the very nature of beauty, which is the normal condition
of a thing being as it should be.
— ADE BETHUNE

So often food was a vehicle for beauty: we set beautiful tables, made tableaus of the food on our plates, or experienced a restaurant as a highly sensory experience. There is nothing wrong with beauty through food, and many of us take daily delight in the rainbow of vegetables we enjoy. But we must be sure that food is not our primary or only avenue to visual pleasure. Perhaps after we are Bright for a while, the calm predictability will bring more order to our physical surroundings and more beauty to our environment. Or we can make space for absorbing beauty through the natural world, through art in all forms, through another's laughter, and through our own moments of clarity.

See if you can expand the avenues by which beauty enters your life. Remember, you do not have to wait until you are in your Bright Body to feel beautiful and share your beauty. You are beautiful!

ON THIS BRIGHT DAY,

I WILL SEEK OUT BEAUTY AND SAVOR WHAT I NOTICE.

April 22

DEPRIVATION

---

*Every man takes the limits of his own field of
vision for the limits of the world.*
— ARTHUR SCHOPENHAUER

Nobody wants to be deprived, but deprivation comes with any diet, which is why none of us can sustain that kind of mindset for the long haul. In BLE, by contrast, we reframe deprivation by focusing on all that we are gaining, even as we no longer eat NMF.

What kind of contentment and inner peace is now available? How did eating NMF or grazing all day long deprive you of *that*? Rather than focusing on what you no longer eat, try leaning into the vast universe of healthy foods, vegetables, grains, proteins, and fruits available to you or perhaps foods or entire sections of the grocery store you overlooked in the past. You will know you have fully inhabited your BLE identity when you do not feel deprived at all while eating—in fact, you are so grateful that you found BLE that you may even consider every mouthful a gift.

ON THIS BRIGHT DAY,

I WILL SEE THE BOUNTY IN MY FOOD AND
IN THE DAY'S EVENTS AS THEY UNFOLD.

April 23

ALLOWING

What the caterpillar calls the end of the world,
the master calls a butterfly.
— RICHARD BACH

Surrender is a popular word for what needs to happen at some point in our journey in order for BLE to be sustainable. However, if using that word conjures up losing in battle, try using *allowing* instead to refer to the portal through which our obsession and food chatter can be lifted.

By allowing the Bright Lines to hold us every single day, our brains heal and those old riverbeds where the waters of addiction once flowed will dry up from disuse. Allowing ourselves to be supported by a loving community means that we are no longer trying to decide everything alone. And allowing ourselves to be fully nourished through connection, as well as healthy food, makes the idea of NMF something fleeting compared to who we are allowing ourselves to be today.

ON THIS BRIGHT DAY,
I WELCOME EVERYTHING THAT HAPPENS,
TRUSTING THAT ALL IS WELL.

ACCEPT JOY

Worry never robs tomorrow of its sorrow,
it only saps today of its joy.
— LEO BUSCAGLIA

Many people think that Bright Line Eating is a body-focused program, but it is really a mind-centric program. Many of us know the experience of crash-dieting down to our goal weight, but because we did not do the inner work on that journey, we were no happier when we saw that magic number on the scale and had no tools to maintain it. So, we started up again with our old patterns of eating, our oldest way to soothe and comfort ourselves.

The key to staying happy once you reach your Bright Body is making sure you feel joy along the way, and all kinds of research indicates that the route to happiness is through connection—with self, with others, and with a higher power or the natural world. Accepting connection as a state of being will allow short-term happiness to ebb and flow, and you won't worry either way because living in connection means knowing all is well and will be well, despite temporary blips. And no blip is so great that it could not be worsened by eating off plan.

ON THIS BRIGHT DAY,

I SEEK CONNECTION AND CULTIVATE JOY.

April 25

BUNNY SLIPPERS

It is in change that things find rest.

— HERACLITUS

In the early days of BLE, you will want to take it easy and give your body plenty of time to detox and recover. We call these "bunny slipper" days. Put your feet up, be gentle with yourself, and do not try to accomplish a lot. This stage does not last forever, and while some of us cannot take time off from parenthood or our jobs, there are discretionary projects and activities that we can ease up on for a while until living the BLE way and using the tools of the program become automatic.

You are taxing your mind with all the preparation and thought that goes into your new way of eating. Give yourself the time and space to do it successfully and you will have a solid foundation from which to launch more projects and be more productive than you have ever dreamed. After your food is automatic, you still need to have an orientation toward life where you allow yourself enough rest when life gets stressful. Even if you have a day stacked with obligations, try to conceive of yourself moving through it with deep breaths, bunny slippers on, and bringing a feeling of ease wherever you go.

ON THIS BRIGHT DAY,

I ALLOW MYSELF THE REST AND SPACE I NEED
TO HOLD MY COMMITMENTS.

April 26
AUTHENTIC SELF

My mother gave me something to live on if she weren't around—spirituality and faith. She gave me her base, her spiritual base, her unshakeable base.

— GLADYS KNIGHT

Our Authentic Self is the pure core of our being. For those with a religious or spiritual tradition, it is through our Authentic Self that we connect with the divine, though the concept of an Authentic Self also transcends any particular spiritual tradition. It simply means that when it comes to knowing what to do next, we have a part of us that knows and wants what is best for ourself.

We know we are in our Authentic Self when we are not judging or anxious and are instead feeling in alignment with the 8 Cs: calm, clear, compassionate, confident, connected, curious, courageous, and creative. Our Authentic Self is separate from the parts that want us to eat more than we need or eat off plan. It is also separate from the parts that are gripping our program so tightly and terrified of deviating in the slightest bit. The Authentic Self energy is not controlling and it is not indulging. It is fully at peace and it can guide us to a Bright Life.

ON THIS BRIGHT DAY,
I WILL TUNE INTO THE CORE OF MYSELF THAT IS
FUNDAMENTALLY UNSHAKEABLE.

MANTRAS

I have suffered enough. That's my favorite mantra
when it comes to motherhood.
— ALI WONG

Mantras are essentially the gatekeepers at the door of our mind, helping us to develop the mental fortitude that it takes to gradually shift from being attached to food as the solution for everything in life to being essentially free from food thoughts. Mantras are phrases that we repeat when we have a spare moment, when we have a food temptation, or when we have a negative thought. They become the natural setting for our mind and give us the nourishing and fortifying thoughts to rest upon when we are idle.

Having phrases that you consciously, intentionally repeat that remind you of your value and keep you within your Bright Lines can be invaluable. Every day of this devotional includes a mantra, but other possible daily mantras include: "That is not my food—that is poison to me," "I am a Bright Lifer," "Nothing tastes as good as keeping my integrity feels," "One day at a time, one meal at a time," "None is easier than some," and "I can do hard things." We serve ourselves well to use a mantra to keep our minds unstoppable.

ON THIS BRIGHT DAY,
I NOTICE MY THOUGHTS AND MAKE A CONSCIOUS
CHOICE FOR POSITIVE INPUT.

April 28
SELF-FORGIVENESS

It is one thing to make the intellectual decision to forgive.
It is another to repeat that decision over and over until it sinks in,
and we begin to feel free from the bondage of our anger.

— MARTHA POSTLETHWAITE

Some of us have withheld forgiveness from ourselves for our years of eating more than our bodies needed, gaining and losing weight through endless dieting, or falling short of other life goals because we were too focused on our weight to have the energy to pursue them. The root of finding self-compassion is to understand that our past selves were doing the best they could at the time with the tools they had.

For some of our wounded inner parts that formed in childhood, self-soothing through food might have been the only tool accessible. As Bright Line Eating opens up access to our Authentic Self, we can now find compassion for the inner parts that were trying to protect us from our wounds—past, present, or future. When we think of it that way, we can find compassion for any part of ourselves.

ON THIS BRIGHT DAY,
I WILL TRY ON THE CLOAK OF FORGIVENESS,
FOR MYSELF AND OTHERS.

HUMOR

Nothing in life is fun for the whole family.
— JERRY SEINFELD

Keeping your sense of humor, especially in the early days of Bright Line Eating, can save your sanity. Food preparation and weighing each meal can feel overwhelming—so much shopping, chopping, and chewing—but they are so important to having a solid foundation for your program. So whenever possible, laugh at the mounds of vegetables. Get giggly if you have accidentally chosen too many light vegetables and are staring down a massive salad. Laugh if you spill your chickpeas or accidentally send a carrot flying. When your humor is gone, your inner Indulger has leverage to get you to eat off plan—and that path isn't *any* fun.

We remember to keep laughing at ourselves and all the ridiculous situations of life because it is the healthy choice . . . and it's fun.

ON THIS BRIGHT DAY,
I WILL LAUGH EASILY AND OFTEN.

THE ISOLATOR

I must admit that I personally measure success in terms
of the contributions an individual makes to her or
his fellow human beings.

— MARGARET MEAD

Addiction loves and requires isolation to thrive, so telling the truth, sharing your vulnerability, and offering support to another can be a game changer when it comes to successfully navigating your life without picking up unplanned food. If you have spent years turning to food instead of turning to people for comfort, support, and guidance, you have got an active Isolator within you that will probably tell you that you do not need other people to work BLE successfully. Do not listen to that. And if you are an introvert, what isolation really means can get quite confusing.

You need ample alone time to recharge and rejuvenate, and taking time for yourself happily and productively is not isolation. Isolation is keeping yourself from support that you need. If you have any sense of loneliness and your Lines are not Bright, you probably need more support than you are allowing yourself.

ON THIS BRIGHT DAY,

I EMERGE FROM ISOLATION TO CONNECT WITH
AND HELP ANOTHER.

May

May 1
FOMO

One doesn't discover new lands without consenting
to lose sight, for a very long time, of the shore.
— ANDRÉ GIDE

When we were eating addictively, we may have felt fear that we would never find a way out of our torment, fear that we would never be able to take care of ourselves the way we wanted to, or fear that we might be eating ourselves into an early grave. Now that we are eating Bright, a new fear may rear its head: Fear of Missing Out. We watch people eating NMF and may feel that our sense of belonging is diminished because we can't participate. We may feel like we attended the wedding, but without the cake, we only experienced part of what everyone else enjoyed.

FOMO is a popular concept right now, but it originates with the neurotransmitter dopamine telling us that there is something better just over the horizon. When it comes to people high on the Food Addiction Susceptibility Scale, though, that horizon is an illusion. What is actually on the other side isn't a greener pasture, but a ditch. What we are missing with BLE pales in comparison to what we are gaining, but if our focus is on what we can't have, we may eventually succumb to temptation.

Better to stay focused on all the gains, the richness and triumph of a life free from the debate over whether or not to eat NMF, and release the fear of missing out.

ON THIS BRIGHT DAY,
I WILL ENJOY WHERE I AM, GIVE MY FULL ATTENTION TO
THE PEOPLE I AM WITH, AND SAVOR THE MOMENT.

May 2

THE KITCHEN IS CLOSED

Success depends upon previous preparation, and without such preparation there is sure to be failure.

— CONFUCIUS

Evenings can be challenging times for overeaters. Putting away leftovers from dinner provides an opportunity for a few Bites, Licks, and Tastes (BLTs), and relaxing with TV or family may historically have been coupled with snacking.

Declaring that the kitchen is closed through some kind of ritual—wiping down the counters and sink, brewing a cup of herbal tea, turning out the lights or shutting the door—can signal to the brain that we are not eating again until breakfast. The time after dinner is also when we begin our Bright tomorrow. It can be productively spent thinking through our next day and preparing, writing down our food, checking our calendar for upcoming appointments, and planning ahead. It is also a great time to make Bright phone calls and connect to our support network. We used to spend evenings numbing ourselves with NMF and mindless entertainment, but today our heart soars with peace and productivity as we use those hours to nourish our Bright Transformation.

ON THIS BRIGHT DAY,

I WILL USE THE TIME AFTER MY THIRD MEAL TO SET MYSELF UP FOR A BRIGHT TOMORROW.

May 3
MASTERMIND GROUP

Spiritual love is a position of standing with one hand extended
into the universe and one hand extended into the world,
letting ourselves be a conduit for passing energy.
— CHRISTINA BALDWIN

We form Mastermind Groups (MMGs) to support our BLE journey. Typically, a group of four to five participants meets weekly (online, via video conference, over the phone, or in person) for roughly 90 minutes. Each person has a chance to check in about their commitment from last week and what they are feeling at the moment, and gets the same number of minutes in the "sweet seat" where they can discuss any issue they would like regarding their BLE program or their life. And each person receives responses of reflection, appreciation, affirmation, or shared experience from the others.

Developing authentic relationships over time through a Mastermind Group means developing new skills, new friendships, and deeper support, all without food. Over the years, we watch as lives ebb and flow and learn one another's patterns, stories, challenges, and triumphs. It is a chance to share what our heart desires with a group that knows and loves us and to have them hold a vision of how we can reach it. Our MMG leaves us inspired.

ON THIS BRIGHT DAY,

I THANK MY MASTERMIND GROUP FOR ITS WISDOM AND
TAKE THE FIRST STEP TO CREATE ONE IF I HAVEN'T YET.

May 4

FIVE-YEAR JOURNAL

A serious life, by definition, is a life one reflects on,
a life one tries to make sense of and bear witness to.
— VIVIAN GORNICK

You are on a remarkable journey of transformation. Why not keep a record of it?

We invite everyone to keep a Five-Year Journal, a format that offers a few lines for each calendar day and has enough space for five years' worth of entries. Because this kind of journal has such a short space in which to write, you will get to winnow and refine what you are recording, noting only highlights, tender moments, or upsetting events. It is an amazing way to track the passage of time.

The events of last year can feel recent, or like they were forever ago. And when we see what happened on that exact day two, three, and then four years ago, we will start to notice seasonal patterns in our life and particular joys and challenges that crop up around annual events. Reading back over the years puts daily events in perspective like nothing else. And noting how far we have come can inspire us to keep striving for better and better tomorrows.

ON THIS BRIGHT DAY,
I BRING MYSELF TO THE PAGE AND REFLECT.

---

100 PERCENT IS EASIER THAN 90 PERCENT

Anytime you see someone more successful than you are,
especially when you're both engaged in the same business,
you know they're doing something that you aren't.

— MALCOLM X

We like to say in BLE that working the program 100 percent is far easier than working it 90 percent, because not breaking any Lines day after day builds the automaticity that allows us to move through the world feeling neutral with food. When our food becomes automatic there is little willpower depletion, and we can rock 100 percent Brightness each day.

On the other hand, breaking our Lines just three days a month means working a 90 percent program. Which is much harder.

Give yourself the gift of 100 percent. If you never make exceptions to the no sugar/no flour Lines, if you weigh and measure exactly without BLTs, and if you eat only during your three mealtimes, you will have *so* much more freedom and ease. Otherwise, you create a brain pathway that allows exceptions and is always on the lookout for the next one. That is not peace.

ON THIS BRIGHT DAY,

I WILL TAKE AN INVENTORY OF MY PROGRAM AND CLOSE
ANY GAP BETWEEN WHAT I AM DOING AND 100 PERCENT.

CREATIVITY

That creative power is in all of you if you give it just a little time;
if you believe in it a little bit and watch it come quietly into you. . . .
— BRENDA UELAND

Little children love to create through imagination and any kind of prop available. But we lose touch with our creativity as we age and start comparing our efforts to others' and judging the outcome. Often overeating tamps down much of our creativity because we can only focus on the next hit.

Once you start on the BLE path, you will find you have more time on your hands and more energy for creative projects. You might return to crafts or hobbies you had abandoned when in the food. Or you might find new ways to use your imagination, your love of beauty, and your skills at building community. Creativity can also find an outlet through playing sports, through entrepreneurship, or even through taking a new route on your daily jog.

Whatever you turn your attention to, let it come from the deepest desires of your heart and watch the food thoughts, temptations, and cravings fade into the background because something bigger and better invites you.

ON THIS BRIGHT DAY,
I WILL LEAN INTO MY CREATIVE IMPULSES.

May 7

WILLINGNESS

Where the willingness is great,
the difficulties cannot be great.
— NICCOLÒ MACHIAVELLI

Willingness is the key to recovery and yet a lot of us do not become willing until we are in an extreme amount of pain. But as we grow in our Bright Journey, we might find that we start to become willing *before* our back is against the wall.

How do you know how willing you are? Talking a good game about keeping your Lines Bright may be a start, but look at your actions too. Is your food planned and prepped? Are your habits strong? Is your support in place? These are the conditions necessary for most of us to stay Bright. It is worth it to find the willingness to work this program. If you find yourself falling off plan, ask yourself what you have been unwilling to do thus far. Then go do that.

There is always another level of action we can take to shore up our program, and if we are resistant, we get curious about it, lean into it, and notice how things change.

ON THIS BRIGHT DAY,
I DISCOVER THE WILLINGNESS WITHIN
TO DO THE TASK BEFORE ME.

HEALING OUR DIGESTION

Make sure that you always follow your heart and your gut,
and let yourself be who you want to be, and who you know you
are. And don't let anyone steal your joy.

— JONATHAN GROFF

Sometimes, after years of eating excess NMF, our guts are compromised. There are those suffering from digestive issues, those who have had bariatric surgery, and those whose digestive system is so unused to raw vegetables that they can initially only consume them cooked. If you have challenges, know that while you are on a Bright Line food plan, the gut typically heals tremendously.

In addition to alleviating tremendous physical discomfort and distress, gut health confers an added benefit to our mental health. Our gut has its own nervous system, and some of our neurotransmitters are found in greater quantities there than in our brain. This scientific awareness gives new depth to the notion of a gut feeling. As we bring our flora back into balance by eliminating white food and empty calories and recolonizing our system with healthy bacteria from raw vegetables, we will gradually feel better—physically *and* mentally. So stay the course knowing that you are healing yourself with every bite.

ON THIS BRIGHT DAY,

I WILL TRUST MY INTUITION AND LISTEN TO MY GUT.

WRITING DOWN OUR FOOD

Commitment is an act, not a word.
— JEAN-PAUL SARTRE

One of the linchpins to developing real peace around food is quieting that part of the brain that says there might be something yummy for us to eat—right now. Writing down our food the night before, even if it is exactly the same menu we had planned for today, builds automaticity and frees us from making food decisions in the moment.

Initially the process can be excruciating for some folks. Yes, we have been there—we have stood over our food journal and taken a long, long time to decide what we are going to eat tomorrow. Still, it is worthwhile, because we do not want a brain that ever asks us, *What would hit the spot right now?*

Once we have written down our food, it is extremely important that we stick to it the next day. Over time, this practice will silence the food chatter in our mind—it will set us free. Also, when we are in the solid habit of writing down our food and it is time to transition to Maintenance, we will benefit because our automaticity is connected to eating what we wrote down, not any specific food plan. This will save us from being tripped up by new amounts, an additional grain, et cetera. Better to have the firm habit of writing down our food so we can let it go and free our mind for other things tomorrow.

ON THIS BRIGHT DAY,
I TAKE THE FUNDAMENTAL ACTIONS THAT ENSURE MY SUCCESS.

HOW SHINY ARE MY LINES?

---

*The truth is too simple: One must always
get there by a complicated route.*

— GEORGE SAND

It is very human to excuse imperfections and rationalize cutting corners. That may be necessary and even healthy in plenty areas of life, but in BLE, our success will be exponentially served by keeping our Lines Bright and 100 percent shiny. The "almost BLE" plan only works if it is working, meaning when we are stable at Maintenance and feeling peaceful. But if our exceptions are escalating or we are regaining significant weight, then it is not working. Then it is time to examine.

Maybe we are eating out more than we need to, choosing restaurants where we know they use a lot of oil in their vegetable preparation. We could shine that up by asking that they steam the vegetables for us. Really. We get to make that request and leave with a shiny Bright Line. If we are feeling overwhelmed, discouraged, or not seeing progress on the scale, we can ask ourselves: *Is our food simple? Are we making exact measurements in every situation?* Ask your Buddy to take a look at your food plan to see where you could tighten things up. You will feel the difference very soon. Promise.

ON THIS BRIGHT DAY,

I WILL RIGOROUSLY LOOK AT HOW I AM
FOLLOWING THE PLAN, NO EXCEPTIONS.

SEE THROUGH THE BITE

There is often in people to whom "the worst" has
happened an almost transcendent freedom,
for they have faced "the worst" and survived it.

— CAROL PEARSON

It can be tempting to romanticize food, imagining eating NMF and drinking NMD, socializing and fitting in, and how delicious and pretty everything looks. But we need to see through that illusion to the next morning, the next month, the next year, to the reality of the bloated stomach, the clothes that don't fit, the increasingly scary bloodwork, the painful joints, and the feelings of depression and desperation.

We know better. We've run the experiment and we know where it leads. So, when your Saboteur tries to paint a pretty picture, drive right through it with your Bright determination. Smash the matrix. See through the seduction and make Bright choices that will create a reality for you that is more wonderful than any fantasy.

ON THIS BRIGHT DAY,

I'LL SEE THROUGH THE FANTASY TO
THE NEW REALITY I'M CREATING.

PAUSE

Many a pair of curious ears had been
lured by that well-timed pause.
— LI ANG

Saying, "No, thank you," to all the possible bites of food in between breakfast, lunch, and dinner requires restraint and the cultivation of a pause that gradually strengthens like a muscle. One of the greatest benefits of staying Bright is the growing ability to take this pause before responding to circumstances.

Without a pause, when life throws us a challenge, we may simply react, and reactions come from old pathways in the brain, old habits formed from traumatic times and stories we have told ourselves for decades. Often these impulses lead us to acts we later regret. But the moment we pause, we have *choice*. We then have a choice about what we eat next, what we say next, and what we put in our shopping carts. Pausing can benefit us in so many areas of life, and that restraint is the beginning of wisdom.

ON THIS BRIGHT DAY,

I PAUSE WHEN I AM UNCERTAIN
AND TAKE A DEEP BREATH
BEFORE SPEAKING OR ACTING.

May 13
RE-CREATION

No entertainment is so cheap as reading,
nor any pleasure so lasting.
— LADY MARY WORTLEY MONTAGU

Research shows that when we work uninterrupted for hours upon hours, our productivity starts to lag. The brain needs breaks. But how often did we use food to provide a break, eating even when we were not hungry because we needed to stop working and did not know how to give ourselves permission without the food?

Food is a poor proxy for real mental replenishment. True recreation nourishes our spirit, refreshes our body, and quiets (or perhaps stimulates) the mind. A brisk walk or a chat with a friend is a far better option for restoring yourself than eating a bag of chips from the vending machine. Breaking for true refreshment and nourishment rather than numbing or distraction offers you the chance to re-create yourself.

Make a list of the activities or non-activities, the spaces, and the people you truly recreate with. Then build that into each day.

ON THIS BRIGHT DAY,
I SET ASIDE TIME TO BE REFRESHED IN WAYS
THAT TRULY NOURISH.

BACK TO BASICS

Not everything that is faced can be changed,
but nothing can be changed until it is faced.
— JAMES BALDWIN

If we slip and need to Rezoom, it is important to review the basics. The Bright Transformation is founded on some simple but profound principles: no sugar, no flour, eat only meals, and weigh and measure our quantities. Write down our food the night before, commit to it, and then the next day eat only and exactly that. Develop a morning routine that we do the same way every day; develop an evening routine to nourish our journey. Connect with and serve others. Those are the fundamentals.

So is your food in order? Have you written it down? Committed it to someone else? Have you prepared food for a day outside the house or done food prep to support you during your upcoming week? Are you performing your morning and evening habit stack? Taking these simple actions can restore the neural pathways and remind yourself, *Oh yes*, this *is who I am.*

ON THIS BRIGHT DAY,

I WILL GET BACK TO BASICS AND DO THE SIMPLE ACTIONS
THAT I KNOW ARE BEST FOR ME.

FOOD CONTROLLER

Possessing a creative mind, after all, is something like
having a border collie for a pet: It needs to work, or else it
will cause you an outrageous amount of trouble.

— ELIZABETH GILBERT

There is a difference between keeping our Lines Bright because our Authentic Self is acting in alignment with our deeply held identity versus our inner Food Controller running the show. Each may result in sticking to the food plan and losing weight, but internally, they feel different. How can we know who is in charge?

If the Food Controller is running your program, you are going to be rigid and perfectionistic with yourself and judgmental and impatient with others when they struggle or break their Lines. If you are working an Authentic Self-Led program, you are going to be compassionate and patient with yourself and others and trust that everyone is on their journey. For most people, it takes a tremendous amount of pain and research and exploration before they really surrender to this way of living.

Compassion, connection, clarity, and curiosity are the hallmarks of the Authentic Self, while judgment, anxiety, fear, and worry are the Food Controller. One is sustainable for a lifetime; the other involves white-knuckling it more than necessary. The route to nourishing our Authentic Self is meditation, creative activities, authentic connection, and moments of gentle rest.

ON THIS BRIGHT DAY,

I WILL RELAX INTO MY AUTHENTIC SELF AND STAY
BRIGHT BECAUSE THIS WAY OF LIFE SERVES ME.

CRAVINGS

The solution is not to combat cravings but to outgrow them.
— OMAR MANEJWALA

Cravings are powerful desires that are created by dopamine downregulation in the mesolimbic reward pathway. However, no matter how strong these urges, they cannot compel us to eat since the mesolimbic pathway does not control our motor coordination.

Think about that. You have another part of your brain, a *higher* part of your brain, that does not have to give in to the craving. Simply knowing that can go a long way toward taking a different action. What you believe about cravings actually affects how you react to them. If you believe you will give in, you do. If you believe that cravings are difficult but you can weather them and let them pass, they do.

The good news is that, as we abstain from sugar and flour, our dopamine receptors repopulate and get more robust, and the overpowering cravings transform into mere passing thoughts.

So there is no reason to be afraid of cravings, but we also should not expect them to dissipate without some action and effort on our part. Once we know they will pass, we take an action to hasten their passage. We pray, breathe for a moment, take a walk, call a friend, get out of the kitchen, use a mantra, start a constructive activity, and get on with our Bright Life.

ON THIS BRIGHT DAY,

I STRENGTHEN MY CONVICTION TO ACT IN MY
BEST INTERESTS, NO MATTER WHAT.

SATIETY

If the only prayer you ever say in your entire life
is thank you, it will be enough.
— MEISTER ECKHART

Satiety comes from the Latin *satis*, meaning "enough." Satiety isn't the feeling of being stuffed; it is the feeling of being at perfect equilibrium. It is the full cup, not the overflowing cup.

Most of us who chronically overate do not know where that zone is. Some of us loved "more" no matter what it was. We loved quantities and that feeling of being overfull, even though our bodies were in a state of distress as our digestive systems harnessed more energy than necessary to break down all of that NMF. Now, in recovery, if we are on the Weight-Loss Food Plan, we eat only enough food to nourish our bodies and lose weight. This, of course, means that our feeling of satisfaction may not last until the next meal.

Simpler foods can leave you more sated because they don't tickle the addiction centers of the brain the way sexy foods do. But hunger may crop up before the next meal. Trusting that hunger is sometimes part of the journey is as important as knowing that your next meal's job is only to get you back to sated. Not stuffed. On our Bright Journey we can relish getting to know our satiety point and trust that our food will always be enough.

ON THIS BRIGHT DAY,
I MARVEL HOW I BRING MYSELF INTO BALANCE
WITH EVERY BRIGHT MEAL.

May 18

TRUE COMFORT

Cure sometimes, treat often, comfort always.

— HIPPOCRATES

Turning to food for comfort is something many of us did as children when human soothing was not sufficient or available. As adults, we can now widen our repertoire of comfort and find out what really soothes our sadness, fills our loneliness, or helps us celebrate our joys. We used food in so many circumstances where we could have done better by ourselves, and now we have the opportunity to seek healthier options.

Take a bubble bath, talk with a friend, read in bed with a hot-water bottle, do a crossword puzzle, or build a fire and watch a great movie. Food as comfort, while socially acceptable, does not work for someone high on the Food Addiction Susceptibility Scale, and when we use food in that way, we will never have enough of what we truly want—which is to ease our emotional suffering. Learning what we do want, what we truly need, is the first step in having that need met. As adults, that is now our job. Nobody can figure it out for us.

ON THIS BRIGHT DAY,

I WILL NOTICE ANY IMPULSE TO EAT THAT COMES UP AND ASK MYSELF WHAT I TRULY WANT.

May 19

A LIFE OF POSSIBILITY

We carry inside us the wonders we seek outside us.
— RUMI

Bright Lifers are frequently amazed at how their lives open once they have decided to follow the program. Yes, weight loss is wonderful and being in a Bright Body allows all kinds of physical activities some of us did not partake in before. But truly the possibilities are endless once the 24-hour obsession with eating, food, weight, size, and debating what choices to make has ended.

The restoration of integrity and trust in ourselves blossoms inside a life that is manageable and well structured and affords us the time to engage in new things and the confidence to take on new roles and responsibilities. When we start to trust ourselves to stay Bright each day, we start to trust ourselves to stretch and grow in life. The life of your dreams is not measured by a clothing size but by positive attitudes about your worth, capability, connections, and contributions.

ON THIS BRIGHT DAY,
I APPRECIATE THE NEW LIFE I AM GROWING INTO
AND THE WONDROUS POSSIBILITIES AHEAD.

UNCERTAINTY

It's hard to face that open space.
— NEIL YOUNG

I t is understandable to have ambivalence about Bright Line Eating. But if you are high on the Food Addiction Susceptibility Scale; if you have tried all kinds of other diets and strategies; or if you are ready for a deep change, better health, and the body you truly want, then stepping up to eat the BLE way is the right next step.

Are you never going to have doubts? Are you never going to look longingly at NMF or NMD ever again? Not likely. But do not give your uncertainty too much attention. Recognize that you do not have to be 100 percent convinced to take the next right action. In fact, we only have to be 51 percent convinced at any given moment to be a 100 percent success. Plenty of Bright Journeys have been successful with deep, deep uncertainty for long stretches.

Acknowledge any uncertainty. One of the most helpful things to do is to talk it through with someone in our community. Because everyone has doubts from time to time, and bringing them out into the light can be a helpful way to stay connected while honoring the part of us that is having doubts. Always make sure you are also looking for evidence of your own success, and that is what you will find.

ON THIS BRIGHT DAY,

I ACKNOWLEDGE ANY DOUBTS AND
MOVE FORWARD ANYWAY.

May 21
PIVOT

Those whom we support hold us up in life.
— MARIE VON EBNER-ESCHENBACH

Pivoting means detaching from a course of action that does not feel right or bring peace and allowing ourselves to be held by a supportive community, a higher power, or our Authentic Self.

Some of us have experienced painful food binges in our life, but there is such a thing as a "mental binge" when negative thoughts develop into a cyclone of toxicity and defeatism that have the capability to knock us out. But even when it feels like we are facing gale-force winds in our mind, we can often just stop them by pivoting away. We say, *No, I am done. I am not going to sink into this.* This 180-degree pivot is firm, like slamming the door on a voice in our brain.

Then there is the much more subtle pivot, the slight shift that opens to a little bit more awareness in the moment, the invitation for grace to come in and a willingness to see a different perspective, to ask: *How could this be happening for me, not to me?* In this way we can pivot away from a food thought or a spiral of negative thinking by unplugging from the emotions or finding the opening for an uplifting thought and a different perspective.

ON THIS BRIGHT DAY,
I TURN AWAY FROM FOOD THOUGHTS AND MENTAL BINGES AND TOWARD THOUGHTS THAT LIFT ME UP.

ORDINARY LIFE

> You *think* there's a joy in a high because it feels good
> temporarily. But it feels good less and less often, so you've
> got to do it more and more often. It ain't your friend.
>
> — WHOOPI GOLDBERG

If you are an intensity junkie, ordinary life can seem boring, and it can be easy to turn to food to punctuate your days with some excitement. Let's face it—the yo-yo dieting days were filled with drama.

One of the addictions we learn to let go of is the need for things to be "interesting" and "different" and "special" all the time. Or even the need to be "busy" and "stressed." Characterizing our lives in that manner can simply be a cortisol addiction that manifests as our brains creating one drama after another to keep life exciting. The truth is, most of our lives are composed of ordinary days, filled with the tasks required to keep life humming. The way to thrive is to pay attention to ordinary times with exquisite attention. When we are present, it is clear that no two moments are exactly the same. And there is tremendous freedom in calm.

ON THIS BRIGHT DAY,

I WILL PAY CAREFUL ATTENTION TO THE
ORDINARY DELIGHTS IN LIFE.

MIND-BODY CONNECTION

It is no use walking anywhere to preach
unless our walking is our preaching.
— ST. FRANCIS OF ASSISI

The mind-body connection has been researched and documented for decades to demonstrate the strong relationship between our thoughts and our health. Research on the placebo effect shows this so powerfully. For example, in a classic Japanese experiment, subjects with an allergy to a specific plant who were blindfolded and told that leaves from that plant were being rubbed on their left arm developed hives, even when the plant was a placebo.[2] The mind is that powerful, which is why things like cravings, food thoughts, and hunger are more under our control than we realize.

Although it can feel like our body is dragging our mind and heart through this enormous challenge of getting sober from sugar and flour, our mind and heart are leading the charge. By aligning them fully and wholeheartedly with our goal, we free our body to release and heal. Our commitment to living Bright can change everything, including how our body experiences our Bright Journey.

ON THIS BRIGHT DAY,

I ALIGN MY THOUGHTS AND ACTIONS TO LIVE IN INTEGRITY.

TRUST THE PLAN

---

*The truth does not change according to our
ability to stomach it emotionally.*

— FLANNERY O'CONNOR

Trust is the keystone of the entryway to a Bright Life. Trust that the plan that has worked for thousands will work for you. Trust that your body will release weight at the rate that is best for your journey. And trust that sticking to the Bright Lines will release the weight, bring you happiness, heal your brain, and afford you levels of freedom you may never have experienced before.

Writing down your food the night before, committing it, and then eating only and exactly that will restore your integrity so that you can again trust yourself. This is so important for those of us who made commitments and promises and then broke them almost daily. Celebrate your growing trust, knowing it is not something that occurs overnight, and keep leaning into that blossoming faith.

ON THIS BRIGHT DAY,

I WILL TRUST THE PLAN AND TRUST MYSELF TO FOLLOW IT,
JUST FOR TODAY.

May 25
SELF-DECEPTION

Secrets are the portal to relapse.
— EARNIE LARSEN

Honesty is the foundation of recovery. But the reality is that we all deceive ourselves, and those of us who are prone to addiction have self-deception woven into the way our brain works. Which most definitely means a history of telling ourselves stories to justify overeating.

The seat of self-deception is known as the Left Hemisphere Interpreter. It notices what we do and spins stories to justify it and does not notice or care if the stories are completely made up. And we believe them. In order to live a Bright Life, we are going to have to examine and reexamine our relationship with our food and learn to get more and more rigorously honest.

Additionally, as we change, we must examine old patterns and images of ourselves that no longer fit. For example, as we lose weight, we may not really see ourselves clearly in the mirror. It takes a long, long time for our self-concept to catch up with our new physical reality. But telling ourselves we are "fat" is a form of self-deception that does not serve us. It can take a while for our eyes to adjust, for us to feel comfortable in our new-sized skin, but listening carefully to the Authentic Self who tells the truth is important. This is the path of integrity: when our body, our mind, and the truth align.

ON THIS BRIGHT DAY,
I WILL NOTICE WHEN I AM NOT BEING HONEST WITH
MYSELF AND ACCEPT THE TRUTH AS IT IS.

FREEDOM

May your life awaken to the call of its freedom.
— JOHN O'DONOHUE

Freedom from and freedom to are two different things. Pay attention to how living the BLE life affords both. Living Bright, you will gain all the benefits of freedom from excess weight and health issues, freedom from mental obsession and endless debate, freedom from self-judgment and condemnation, freedom from regret and remorse.

But also notice the more subtle freedoms you are gaining access to: freedom to be more creative, freedom to have greater intimacy, freedom to choose how you spend your time, and freedom to take exceptional care of your body.

The Bright Lines, by their very nature, are constraints and that can feel confining at times, but upon deeper reflection we relish and appreciate all the gifts of freedom our commitment to this way of living affords us.

ON THIS BRIGHT DAY,
I CELEBRATE THE FREEDOM I ENJOY BY LIVING BRIGHT.

SIGNIFICANT SHIFTS

Progress is impossible without change, and those who cannot
change their minds cannot change anything.
— GEORGE BERNARD SHAW

Sometimes we can have a moment of clarity and a powerful inner shift of surrender and willingness all at once. Or we can stick with the plan day in and day out and then lose a startling amount of weight in what seems like a very short period of time. Or we can do some inner work and have an awareness that changes our reaction to a family member or significant person in our life and our experience in that relationship shifts quickly and dramatically. But other times the changes are incremental and subtle.

BLE creates significant changes in our lives. We call these transformations Non-Scale Victories (NSVs). And NSVs can happen incrementally—or instantaneously. They often only reveal themselves upon reflection. We can pay attention to these shifts by building in daily reflection time, using our five-year journal, or inviting someone who knows us well to share how we have changed—they may see what we cannot. We are often surprised at the differences that gradually occur as we live the BLE way.

ON THIS BRIGHT DAY,

I NOTICE AND CELEBRATE MY INCREMENTAL PROGRESS.

May 28

JUST RESET

Where would the gardener be if there were no more weeds?
— CHUANG TZU

If we have had a break in our Lines, it is important to reset quickly. We can reset our day at any point rather than waiting until tomorrow, or Monday, or next January. We can start again right now by having an attitude reset. *That was the past. This is now. I am not beholden to that old behavior, and I get to do something different in this moment.* The present is the point of choice, and it's the place where we set our intention to act differently.

This does not just apply to the food. If we are frustrated with our kids or our partner, if we are engaged in really harmful self-talk, if we are procrastinating and avoiding a task we really need to be doing, we can just stop and reset. Resetting creates the foundation to act the way we would like to, starting now.

ON THIS BRIGHT DAY,

I WILL NOTICE A MOMENT WHERE I AM OFF TRACK,
STOP, AND RESET.

FUN

> I cannot even imagine where I would be today
> were it not for that handful of friends
> who have given me a heart full of joy.
> — CHARLES R. SWINDOLL

As adults, we can forget about the importance of having fun. Sadly, a lot of us have come to live without silliness, laughter, play, and adventure. Which has led some of us to use food to have fun. That is understandable as food is at the center of so much celebration, bonding, and socializing. However, learning to have fun without food becomes a crucial skill.

So today, think about what is fun for you. Is it laughing? Then pull up a humorous clip on YouTube. Dancing? Go put on some music and groove in the shower. Pickleball? Get online and find a local team. Playing board games? Invite some friends over for a game night. Rolling around with your dog? Make time for a walk that allows for some unstructured play.

Fun is not superfluous. It is important for infusing our days with joy and elevating our spirits. It creates lasting memories and puts the *bright* in our Bright Journey.

ON THIS BRIGHT DAY,

I INFUSE SOME FUN INTO MY DAY.

CROSS-ADDICTION

More, Now, Again . . .

— ELIZABETH WURTZEL

How many times have we given up one addiction only to find our addictive urges popping up somewhere else? Shopping more, flirting incessantly, or spending more time on our screens? When we take away the sugar and flour, the addiction centers in our brain will look elsewhere for that dopamine hit and we can find ourselves gambling, shopping, smoking pot, smoking cigarettes, vaping, drinking lots of coffee, or even drinking can after can of sparkling water.

It is easy to substitute a new addiction if we don't do the inner work required to be comfortable with ourselves as we are. The real path of recovery is to let go of abusing *anything*. The invitation is to make friends with the emptiness after the food is removed. Recovery is a long journey. Sometimes we will be willing to see the new addiction and nip it in the bud. Sometimes willingness will take time. Along the way we can give ourself the gift of noticing, staying tuned in to our Authentic Self, and listening.

ON THIS BRIGHT DAY,

I WILL BE AWARE OF OTHER ADDICTIONS AND EMBRACE
A WHOLEHEARTED JOURNEY OF RECOVERY.

May 31
PLATEAUS

Facing it, always facing it, that's the way to get through. Face it.
— JOSEPH CONRAD

Plateaus in our weight-loss journey can be frustrating, yet often people declare one sooner than necessary. Our Lines have to be shiny Bright and our weight stable for several months in order to officially be on a plateau.

Often plateaus are caused by small actions that we don't realize can prevent forward progress, like using supplement powders or condiments, roasting our vegetables with lots of spray oil, or not being mindful enough in restaurants, even if it is just one or two restaurant meals per week. If we think our weight has plateaued, we can scale back on condiments, avoid eating out, steam our vegetables for a while and see if that moves the needle. We can also make sure we are staying active with NEAT, which stands for non-exercise activity thermogenesis. The easiest way to do that is to get a step counter and aim for 10,000 steps a day.

If we do this inventory and find that no adjustments are required, then we must trust that our body is taking exactly the time it needs to let us get caught up with our new size.

ON THIS BRIGHT DAY,
I TRUST MY MOMENTUM BY FOLLOWING
THE BLE PLAN EXACTLY.

June

June 1
SISU

Grit is living life like it's a marathon, not a sprint.
— ANGELA DUCKWORTH, PH.D.

In our Bright Journey, there may be days when we are white-knuckling our way from meal to meal, when every hour we manage to not succumb to NMF is a major victory. The Finnish word *sisu* describes the qualities of tenacity, persistence, and bravery that the Finnish people called upon when they beat the odds to defeat the Russian army in the Winter War of 1939–40. Modern psychologists, led by Angela Duckworth, use the term "grit" to define the passion and perseverance for long-term goals. In BLE, we invoke the concepts of grit and sisu to keep us focused on our long-term goals and remind ourselves that no matter how deep the old neural pathways are that tell us to eat when life gets hard, we have the inner strength to do something different.

Every day we call upon that courage and bravery to reach out for support, write about what we are feeling, drink a cup of herbal tea, and stay strong until our next Bright meal is a victory. We are unstoppable.

ON THIS BRIGHT DAY,
I WILL DRAW UPON MY INNER RESOURCES.

June 2

JUST GO TO BED

At the end of the day, the goals are simple: safety and security.

— JODI RELL

When we first get sober from food addiction and start eating three meals a day at regular mealtimes, our peripheral clock—the cells in our digestive system, liver, and kidneys that are keeping track of time—align with our central clock (the SCN or suprachiasmatic nucleus) in our hypothalamus. Our circadian rhythm becomes much stronger, meaning we sleep better, and we tend to go to sleep earlier, both because we run out of fuel and because we are not reprogramming our system with late-night eating and cueing it to think it should be alert into the wee hours. Our systems are designed to take in fuel only when the sun is up, so this is a healthy, natural part of the daily rhythm of Bright Line Eating.

If getting through the day starts to feel hard, we end the day by just going to bed. The deep rest and safety of our bed, far from the kitchen, restores us, and an early bedtime sets us up for a Bright tomorrow.

ON THIS BRIGHT DAY,

I TREAT MYSELF TO AN EARLY BEDTIME.

CONTENTMENT

When one's thoughts are neither frivolous nor flippant,
when one's thoughts are neither stiff-necked nor stupid,
but rather, are harmonious—they habitually render
physical calm and deep insight.

— HILDEGARD OF BINGEN

Our brains were not designed for contentment; they were designed to scan the environment and assess, *What is wrong? What needs to be changed? Where am I in danger?* This negativity bias was critical when our species was living in the wild and survival was challenging. However, today it can mean that those of us who are prone to dopamine dominance have a brain that is constantly dissatisfied.

Contentment is a quieter state of being, though it requires some fine-tuned attention to be aware of it. To nurture contentment, we must become more awake to the present moment. Neurotransmitters like oxytocin and serotonin will help, and the daily pattern of living Bright encourages our brains to replenish them as we let go of the excess stimulation of sugar and flour. Make a decision to be content, and be astonished at all the ways life conspires to make you happy.

ON THIS BRIGHT DAY,

I WILL NOTICE A MICRO-MOMENT OF
CONTENTMENT AND SAVOR IT.

CLARITY

Clarity of vision is the key to achieving your objectives.
— TOM STEYER

Mental clarity is not typically the first benefit people have in mind when they start BLE. This is predominantly due to the fact that it is impossible to fully perceive the mental fog that a diet of sugar and flour and processed foods creates when we have lived inside it for years. It is only when those substances are cleared from our body that we recognize what mental clarity and agility feel like.

Fueling our day with caffeine and sugar and processed foods creates a lot of unmanageability and chaos. As we weigh and measure our food, we start to weigh and measure our lives. And as we clear the sugar and flour and processed foods out of our brain, integrity with our food choices creates integrity with how we are living. Life comes into crisp focus and we can move forward with confidence.

ON THIS BRIGHT DAY,
I ENJOY WATCHING MY LIFE COME INTO FOCUS.

REPETITION

Boredom is rage spread thin.
— PAUL TILLICH

The key to success in recovery is repetition. Addicts by their very nature seek a lot of stimulation, and excess is baked into the problem. In sobriety we learn to eschew that kind of toxic excitement through humbled repetition. We repeat our morning habits, we repeat our evening pattern, we repeat our service calls, and we retrain our brain not to seek so much variation. And some of us find value in eating the same thing every day, especially when we are first healing.

If you love variety in your food and get bored quickly with the same breakfast, lunch, or dinner, it might be worth examining what needs you are trying to fulfill through your food choices. Conversely, do not apologize if you eat the same thing regularly. Some of the most successful people in BLE eat the same foods every day to eliminate the need for decisions, choices, and entertainment. They then turn their attention and energy into having variety and diversity in other arenas of life.

ON THIS BRIGHT DAY,
I WILL SEE THE RICHNESS IN ROUTINE.

MORNING RITUALS

The human soul can always use a new tradition.
Sometimes we require them.

— PAT CONROY

Early morning, possibly even before anyone else in our household is awake, is the time of day when we have the most control to craft our habits. Once the day is underway, our time can slip out of our grasp. Meditating, journaling, praying, absorbing a page from this devotional, writing a gratitude list, prepping lunch (and perhaps dinner), reaching out to a Buddy, checking in with the online community—these are all foundational activities that remind us of our BLE identity and reinforce it before we have even had a single bite to eat.

Every morning that we follow through on our morning routine we are telling ourselves, *I am a Bright Lifer. I do not eat sugar or flour. I eat three meals a day and nothing in between. I weigh my portions.* A day started well is a day we are likely to succeed.

Think of what nourishes you more deeply than excess food and put that into your morning habit stack. And if you need to get to bed earlier to give yourself the gift of those precious morning minutes to center, we invite you to explore that too.

ON THIS BRIGHT DAY,

I GLADLY PERFORM THE HABITS THAT
SET ME UP FOR SUCCESS.

MOVEMENT

There are shortcuts to happiness,
and dancing is one of them.
— VICKI BAUM

BLE takes the radical stance that, in general, starting to exercise is not helpful in the first few months of the program. Too much willpower is depleted forcing ourselves to move when we need to use every ounce of our reserves to eat only and exactly what we have committed to eat.

But once our brain has healed and our leptin is registering in the hypothalamus again, we will feel a desire to start moving. Gentle stretching and easy walks are a great beginning, provided they are not stressful and do not require harnessing our will to accomplish them. But if we were folks who mainly went from the bed to the table to the car to the chair and back again, once we have been Bright for a few months, we know we really must try to get in movement throughout the day. We learn to take the stairs at work, walk to the store, vacuum instead of turning on the Roomba—it all adds up. And once we reach Maintenance, we have a strong foundation and excellent habits supporting us, and before we know it, we find that our regular exercise routine is simply a joy.

ON THIS BRIGHT DAY,

I NOTICE WHAT MOVEMENT MY BODY WANTS
AND GENTLY LEAN INTO IT.

MEDICATION CHANGES

Science is really in the business of disproving current models
or changing them to conform to new information. In essence,
we are constantly proving our latest ideas wrong.

— DAVID SUZUKI

As we begin our Bright Line Journey, even before we have lost much weight, our blood work will change. Triglycerides will go down, insulin sensitivity will begin to be restored, blood pressure will improve. All of that will require the re-dosing of medications for cholesterol, high blood pressure, diabetes, and more, so we are careful to stay in close contact with our health care provider as we lose weight. Additionally, changing body weight affects dosage, and few in the health professions realize how fast someone can lose weight following a food plan that contains no sugar and flour. They will not be able to predict our rate of weight loss, so it is our responsibility to keep them informed. Furthermore, since sugar is depressive and vegetable consumption correlates with vibrant mental health, some psychiatric medications may need to be adjusted or tapered as well. On our Bright Journey we stay in tune with our changing chemistry and in touch with our health care providers as our bodies and brains heal.

ON THIS BRIGHT DAY,

I TAKE THE ACTIONS THAT SUPPORT MY CHANGING
BRAIN AND BLOOD CHEMISTRY.

GRATITUDE JOURNAL

I think true gratitude involves a humble dependence on others:
We acknowledge that other people—or even higher powers,
if you're of a spiritual mindset—gave us many gifts, big and small,
to help us achieve the goodness in our lives.

— ROBERT EMMONS

Myriad studies demonstrate that gratitude has a powerful positive impact on our brain. It can make us less depressed and less anxious while also improving our immune system and our health. But we have to keep it fresh. We want many other aspects of our BLE program to become automatic, but not our gratitude, because then it becomes mindless and not in a good way. So, find different ways to engage with your gratitude journal. Write down "A–Z" and find something for each letter. Pick the hardest challenge in your life and brainstorm everything you are grateful for about it (so beneficial!). Write 10 big things you are grateful for and 10 tiny things. Because if you want contentment, focus on gratitude. If you want ease in your day, be sure to appreciate what you can do. If you want healthier relationships, be grateful for the good qualities in those around you. Consciously adding to your happiness by writing down what has worked today, what has been joyful, or where you have felt content—what some might call blessed—is a powerful tool.

ON THIS BRIGHT DAY,
I WILL FIND NEW THINGS TO APPRECIATE.

June 10
STRETCH YOURSELF

---

*What's terrible is to pretend that the second-rate is first-rate.
To pretend that you don't need love when you do; or you like your
work when you know quite well you're capable of better.*
— DORIS LESSING

There is a saying that goes, "The person I was will always eat, so I have to change." BLE is a grand experiment in changing how you eat, of course. But it is also an experiment in creating new habits, making new connections, and getting to know yourself more intimately than ever before. Try all the tools to see which ones are most helpful to you. Reach out to all kinds of people, not just those who seem most like you. When Susan Peirce Thompson first stopped using drugs, she was told to ask God to keep her clean and sober each day. She just laughed and said, "I don't believe in God." They said, "Well, have you ever prayed?" When she said no, they asked, "Well, are you a scientist or aren't you? Run the experiment." So she tried praying every morning and after a few months she became aware that it was working—the obsession to use drugs had been lifted. You never know what might work unless you try it. Stretch yourself to be of service way before you think you are ready, and you will find yourself in new territory with a kind of aliveness you may have never thought possible.

ON THIS BRIGHT DAY,
I WILL LOOK FOR OPPORTUNITIES TO GET OUT
OF MY COMFORT ZONE.

BUILD FORWARD MOMENTUM, NOT SPEED

When the doors of promise open,
the trick is to quickly walk through them.

— GORDON PARKS

The Bright Transformation celebrates the life that we get to live right here, right now. Which is why when it comes to weight-loss rates, it is irrelevant that some people lose more rapidly than others. The point is not the speed but the forward momentum. If the scale is going down, celebrate that rather than berate it for not being fast enough. If you are feeling more days of contentment, take note of that rather than complain about the challenging days. If you can focus on what is working, you can add to the momentum of your Bright Transformation. If you take score of where you are and compare it to another or some hypothetical ideal, you will slow your momentum. The idea that there is somewhere to rush to is treating this as a diet, and it is not a diet, it is a lifestyle. The people who are successful with BLE long term settle into the weight-loss phase as if it is forever. In Maintenance, that forward momentum translates to growth and increased effectiveness in our relationships and our quality of life. Here is the great news: wherever you are, you have already arrived.

ON THIS BRIGHT DAY,

I FOCUS ON THE JOURNEY, NOT THE DESTINATION.

June 12

RESTLESSNESS

Anxiety is the gap between the now and the later.
— FRITZ PERLS

Restlessness is a red flag in BLE because it is usually a sign of dopamine downregulation, which can last for some time after sugar and flour are removed from the diet. When addicts need a hit, the feeling is one of restlessness—itchy irritability that drives them to get relief. While we wait for the brain to heal, we may feel bored with our food and tired of having to weigh it, annoyed by coaching calls, or isolated from others. These old feelings used to be soothed by food, and now we have to use a different tool to help ourselves. If you are feeling restless with your progress or if you find yourself snapping at others or silently judging everyone and everything that crosses your path, take that as a sign that you need more support, more connection, and perhaps even more depth to your life. Sit with it, lean into it, and get curious about what is really going on. The still, small voice deep inside may surprise you with a nudge to do something that is the next step for you.

ON THIS BRIGHT DAY,

I WILL PAUSE WHEN FEELING RESTLESS AND
BRING MY ATTENTION TO THIS PRECIOUS MOMENT.

June 13

RISK

Only those who are being burned know what fire is like.
— ETHEL WATERS

What is the risk of getting sober from sugar and flour? Old patterns are disrupted, and we might have to face a lot of feelings of discomfort. We might even be confronted by old traumas that need to be healed. Then there is the risk of failure; the part of us that has been so hurt by failures in the past might not want us to take that risk. What is the risk if you do not commit to BLE? You may never know what it feels like to be in a Bright Body, to have the best health you can possibly achieve, and to feel free from food obsession, chatter, and temptation. If you do not give it your all, you risk never knowing what it feels like to break free. It is your choice which risk you want to take—but there is risk on both sides because we are talking about your body and your soul. Where the stakes are high, so will be the risk.

ON THIS BRIGHT DAY,
I TAKE A RISK TO DO WHAT IS NEEDED FOR MY SUCCESS.

FRIENDSHIP

Love and compassion are necessities, not luxuries.
Without them humanity cannot survive.
— DALAI LAMA

At BLE we encourage people to seek support from others in the program. Whether it is a daily phone call with a Buddy, a weekly walk with someone in the program, a regular Mastermind Group call, or all three, these conversations are an invaluable source of unconditional support. Many people are not used to being so supported, held, understood, and affirmed, and BLE becomes a breeding ground for real friendships. Because at some point you stop talking about food and start talking about life.

When you invest in friendship with other Bright Lifers by sharing your own struggles, authentically showing up for them, and loving them under all conditions, you create a strong network of support that will hold you when life gets challenging. The fellowship of the BLE network, the unconditional love that is given and received, and the deep affection we have for those around the world who are living the BLE life is one of the greatest gifts.

ON THIS BRIGHT DAY,

I WILL BE AS COMPASSIONATE AND LOVING AS
POSSIBLE AND NOTICE THE GIFTS THAT COME TO ME
BECAUSE OF THAT ATTITUDE.

June 15

FOCUS ON WHAT IS WORKING

Hope is a song in a weary throat.
— PAULINE MURRAY

There are a lot of moving parts in a full recovery program to keep you nourished so you do not turn to NMF—food plans and commitments, morning and evening habit stacks, phone calls and support in good times so it is just what you do in hard times. These all take energy, and putting each one in place is an accomplishment. Sometimes we can get too focused on the aspects of the journey that feel wobbly, be it our rate of weight loss, tenacious body image issues, or difficulty in letting go of NMF. But attention is a form of nourishment, so focusing on what *is* working will help bring what is wobbly into alignment. What you focus on expands, and although we are hardwired to pay attention to what is amiss, we have to discipline ourselves to see what is working. Spend a week not complaining about anything and watch your happiness rise. Focus on what your children do well and watch their behavior improve. Shower your partner with appreciation and watch them blossom. Do the same with your own self-talk and watch your BLE program get easier.

ON THIS BRIGHT DAY,

I FOCUS ON WHAT IS WORKING AND WHAT
FILLS ME WITH PRIDE AND HOPE.

June 16

COURAGE

Never bend your head. Always hold it high.
Look the world straight in the eye.
— HELEN KELLER

The root of courage comes from the French word for heart: *couer*. To be courageous means living a wholehearted life, jumping in with both feet, saying the whole truth, and sharing your whole self—insecurities, arrogance, and everything in between. It requires courage to do something so countercultural as to not eat sugar and flour. To be willing to face difficult emotions that you have eaten over for a lifetime. To advocate for yourself in restaurants, family gatherings, and the workplace break room. Take stock of how courageous you have been on this journey. Honor that part of you that is capable of more than you realized and welcome the next opportunity to expand your capacity to speak, live, and decide from your heart.

ON THIS BRIGHT DAY,
I WILL LIVE WHOLEHEARTEDLY AND ACKNOWLEDGE
THE COURSE IT TAKES TO STAY TRUE TO MY CONVICTIONS.

LIGHT-UP FOODS

Sometimes you just gotta trust that your
secret's been kept long enough.
— ANNE CAMERON

Not all BLE foods are created equal. Many of the foods on the list of acceptable BLE foods are quite simple: vegetables, fruits, simple proteins. Other foods are more processed, like flour-free crackers, nut butters, and cheese. You get to try all the foods in all the categories of the BLE food plan. But you also get to notice if there are some foods that light you up; foods you find yourself looking forward to, feeling too attached to, or scared to take out of your food plan; or foods that you have a history of bingeing on, even if they are BLE-compliant. There may be some BLE foods you simply cannot keep in your home. That is okay. You will not go hungry, because there are many foods you can eat safely and never feel tempted to indulge. Recognizing foods that light you up requires rigorous honesty with yourself, and time out from them may be a gift you give yourself for a while. This break will allow a deeper level of healing for your brain and spirit.

ON THIS BRIGHT DAY,
I WILL TELL SOMEONE ABOUT THE
FOODS THAT LIGHT ME UP.

TRUE ENTERTAINMENT

We do not cease to play because we grow old.
We grow old because we cease to play.
— GEORGE BERNARD SHAW

How often was food the centerpiece of a social gathering, the very reason to get together? How often did some form of NMF "make" the occasion? How often did you buy NMF when seeing a movie, or eat NMF when you watched TV? When you no longer make food the centerpiece of social connection, you give yourself a chance to discover what really does refresh and entertain you. Many successful Bright Lifers discover hobbies they have always wanted to try but did not have time for in their food-obsessed days. Others rediscover a love of music, gardening, crafts, or writing that went by the wayside as their health deteriorated. Others are at a time of life when playing on the floor with grandchildren or children becomes something they now can do without hesitation. On this Bright Journey, we enjoy finding out what really interests us without the crutch of NMF and we cultivate those conversations, connections, and activities.

ON THIS BRIGHT DAY,

I APPROACH THE WORLD WITH THE WONDER
OF THE CHILD WITHIN ME.

NEW IDENTITY

---

*When people get married because they think
it's a long-time love affair, they'll be divorced very soon,
because all love affairs end in disappointment.
But marriage is a recognition of a spiritual identity.*

— JOSEPH CAMPBELL

To succeed with Maintenance, we must shift our identity to someone who has *arrived* and truly let go of the food and the weight struggle. That means being willing to stop tinkering with our weight range, let go, and surrender to the reality that the problem has been solved. We do not need to strive or struggle anymore. The next invitation is to be willing to face the fear of the vacuum that has now been created in our life. It feels scary to not organize our life around our food struggles. There is a part of us that wants to avoid the empty space.

Our new challenge is to fill our life with other things, other interests, and a new identity. Bright Line Eating provides so much of that new identity through friendships and community. But know that you are embarking on a period of exploration as you meet this new surrendered self.

ON THIS BRIGHT DAY,

I AM OPEN TO MY NEW IDENTITY.

ENDINGS

If you let yourself be absorbed completely,
if you surrender completely to the moments as they pass,
you live more richly those moments.
— ANNE MORROW LINDBERGH

Closure can be an important ritual that signifies the end of one identity, phase, or cycle and the birth of a new one. There are plenty of endings in BLE. In the early days of BLE, we say good-bye to many of the foods that we thought were our friends, until we learned that they had been sabotaging our health and happiness. Grieving those foods—writing a letter of good-bye to the old self who ate addictively or to the specific binge foods we were most attached to—can be a useful exercise.

We eventually end the weight-loss phase and move into Maintenance, where the thrill of seeing the scale go down has to be transferred to the more subtle satisfaction of never seeing it go up rapidly again. This ending too requires attention and care. We had become attached to the security of the Weight-Loss Food Plan, and adding food feels scary.

Unlike in the days when we ate through all transitions and somewhat sleepwalked through life, we strive to stay aware of endings. This helps with the transition to the next chapter and living that consciously helps us feel more alive.

ON THIS BRIGHT DAY,

I ACCEPT THE BITTERSWEETNESS THAT MAY COME
WITH ENDINGS AS I AWAIT A NEW BEGINNING.

COMMITMENT

There is no such thing as freedom without discipline.
The one who is free is disciplined.
— JANET COLLINS

All of us make a commitment to BLE at the beginning that propels us to do the hard work of creating a solid foundation for our program, so that eventually it becomes so automatic it is just the way we live. But as we move along on our journey, there are deeper commitments asked of us. We commit to being fully courageous and getting extra support when we transition into Maintenance. Finally, there is a commitment to serving the BLE community, to helping others who are starting out, struggling, or ready to quit. With our deep commitment we become a shining example for those in our life, without preaching or giving advice, of the ease and success of BLE. That commitment to the best in ourself, to keeping integrity by keeping our Lines Bright, begins to be the new set point for our emotions and discipline, and it all starts by turning fully in the direction of what we want and committing to do whatever it takes today to stay there.

ON THIS BRIGHT DAY,

I ALLOW MY COMMITMENT TO CARRY ME ACROSS
THE THRESHOLD OF RESISTANCE.

June 22

RESPECT

*I am only really myself when I'm somebody
else whom I have endowed with these wonderful
qualities from my imagination.*

— ZELDA FITZGERALD

Respect can be a guidepost in our recovery. When it comes to our self-respect, eating the BLE way certainly demonstrates that, but what other areas of our program could be strengthened by active respect? Are we respecting our mealtimes and our food? Are we keeping our Lines crisp with no Bites, Licks, and Tastes? Are we not putting anything in our mouth until we sit down at the table, take a breath, and feel a moment of humble gratitude that we made it to the table for yet another Bright meal? Motivational speaker Jim Rohn famously said that you become the average of the five people you spend the most time with. With that in mind, look around at who you are hanging out with in Bright Line Eating. Do you respect the program they are working, and how they treat themselves in this program? What qualities do you admire or respect in a person? Are you surrounding yourself with people who embody those qualities? Do you admire them? Do you want to be more like them? When we respect the program and the people we walk alongside, we respect and honor ourself.

ON THIS BRIGHT DAY,

I RESPECT MY PROGRAM AND LOOK FOR
THAT QUALITY IN OTHERS.

MECHANISTIC OR HOLISTIC

Life is a process of becoming, a combination
of states we have to go through. Where people fail
is that they wish to elect a state and remain in it.

— ANAÏS NIN

Our bodies are not machines. While BLE sets out guidelines that work for nearly everyone, there may be subtle shifts or timetables that remain mysterious regarding weight loss (or gain). The reality is that psychology, social factors, and biology interact in very complex ways. One example that we see repeatedly is the subtle way that our bodies let us know that they do or do not trust us. Oftentimes, people who have been slightly dishonest with their food (though in a calorically negligible way) find that when they finally surrender their addictive eating on a deeper level, they suddenly release their excess weight. This is a psychological shift, a spiritual shift, if you will. Taking a holistic, gentle, long-term approach will serve you much better than assuming that because you are eating only and exactly what is on your food plan you should lose weight at a certain rate or maintain a specific goal weight. Holistic approaches take into account social support, emotional balance, and spiritual health—the whole wonderful you.

ON THIS BRIGHT DAY,

I HAVE RESPECT FOR ALL THE FACTORS THAT
PLAY INTO MY PROGRAM AND THE WAY
THAT THEY INTERACT AND INTERTWINE.

PATIENCE IS KEY TO SUSTAINABILITY

I change myself, I change the world.
— GLORIA ANZALDÚA

Too often we expect the scale to move immediately once we have made a change in our food plan. But impatience is the hallmark of diet mentality. And diets do not get us anywhere. We have had enough of the yo-yo cycle of rapid weight loss followed by weight regain and disillusionment. In recovery, patience and trust are the key to sustainability. We have to be in this for the long haul or it is nothing more than a temporary diet.

When we are frustrated with our progress on the scale, we remind ourselves that even small weight losses compounded over time equals a Bright Transformation. The years will pass anyway; when we are Bright, we are on the right path. Acknowledging that this process does not happen overnight and our weight will not be reversed in an instant is key to shifting our attention from results to enjoying every day on the way. You can't get to happy on an unhappy road.

ON THIS BRIGHT DAY,
I SETTLE IN, HAVE PATIENCE,
AND ENJOY THE JOURNEY.

BROKEN EYES

When we are chafed and fretted by small cares,
a look at the stars will show us
the littleness of our own interests.
— MARIA MITCHELL

Even after losing many pounds, some people look in the mirror and see their old self. If you have broken eyes, you may still assume you are the largest person in the room, worry about chairs holding you, or fear getting on an airplane because you will need a seatbelt extender. Then there are those of us who get dangerously underweight and think that we still have yet more weight to lose. Body dysmorphia is rampant in communities of people who have an addictive relationship with food.

The reality is that it is not our body that needs to be fixed, but the glasses through which we are seeing our body. If we are looking through glasses of dissatisfaction, we will always be dissatisfied, period. No matter how much weight we lose, it takes time to see ourselves clearly and maybe even more time to release the judgment about how we look. Because even at our heaviest, we were good, worthy, loveable people. And that is what we hope to see today when we look in the mirror, regardless of our size.

ON THIS BRIGHT DAY,

I LET GO OF BODY OBSESSION AND
FOCUS ON MY HAPPINESS.

June 26
LARGER PURPOSE

The place God calls you is where your deep gladness
and the world's deep hunger meet.
— FREDERICK BUECHNER

Losing weight and being in a Bright Body is not an end unto itself, but rather a means to doing what you would like to do with your life. If losing weight is the whole point, you will likely regain weight in order to lose it again. You must have a larger purpose for being that is enhanced by a healthier body, because pursuing peak fitness or beauty is a distraction. The goal is really peace and freedom from the food chatter so that we can live into our larger purpose. That is what the whole Bright Line Eating movement is about: releasing all that human potential that is trapped, not just underneath the weight, but underneath the obsession with the weight. To hit the ground running at Maintenance, it is important to internalize that living in a Bright Body can be useful for moving comfortably in the world, but the deeper gift is being able to hear where you are being called to, where your unique gifts and talents are going to be most useful. *This* is the deep work that accompanies weight loss.

ON THIS BRIGHT DAY,

I GENTLY LEAN INTO WHAT VIBRATES MY SOUL.

SELF-APPRECIATION

---

*If you regularly rest your mind upon . . . noticing
you're all right right now, seeing the good in yourself, and
letting go . . . then your brain will gradually take the
shape of calm strength, self-confidence, and inner peace.*

— RICK HANSON

It is an honoring, affirming exercise to take a friend or a child—someone close in our life—and sit down to study and appreciate them. To not be able or willing to do the same for ourselves is a false form of humility. The gap between our ability to do that for another and do it for ourselves is a measure of inner work that is left to be done. Do not wait until you have lost weight to appreciate yourself. The fine qualities you have are present today, and the sooner you can acknowledge, access, and affirm them, the happier you will be and the easier it will be to stick to your Bright Lines. Because those with a sense of self that is rooted in compassion do better things for themselves. Nobody makes lasting changes because they have been judged or criticized. It is love and seeing the best in ourselves that elicits transformation. We all see the wonder of you! Won't you take the time to appreciate yourself today? Make a list of your positive attributes, look for evidence of your goodness, and amaze yourself.

ON THIS BRIGHT DAY,

I WILL INVENTORY WHAT I LOVE ABOUT MYSELF.

June 28

BUFFERING

The biggest enemies of willpower:
temptation, self-criticism, and stress.
— KELLY MCGONIGAL

Willpower gets depleted with every decision we make, every stressor we navigate, every challenge we encounter. And when our willpower is depleted, absolutely everything feels overstimulating. Loud sounds get louder. Annoyances feel more annoying. It is as if we are protected under a cozy blanket and when our willpower is depleted, the blanket becomes threadbare and the cold and wind and noise come through. Research offers us ways to reinforce our blanket each day, through meditation, gratitude, prayer, journaling, seeking social support, being in the natural world, playing and having unscheduled time, doing for others, and getting enough sleep. All of these will keep you nicely buffered with willpower so that when additional stressors are added they won't ruffle you.

ON THIS BRIGHT DAY,

I WILL INTENTIONALLY CONNECT WITH NOURISHING
PEOPLE TO REPLENISH MY WILLPOWER.

June 29
SET ASIDE

Knowing others is wisdom;
knowing the self is enlightenment.

— LAO TZU

Expertise can obviously be valuable in many fields, but so often our preconceptions are our limiting factor. If you bring old beliefs about how weight loss works, how you will do, or what is possible, you will unnecessarily limit your experience in BLE. It is beginner's mind that has the most possibilities for contentment, especially at the start of something. Setting aside what you think you know can open the mind to new ideas, new approaches, and more nuanced understandings. In the trust fall, you fold your arms into your chest, stand stiff as a board, and fall backward into the arms of waiting friends. Setting aside our preconceptions is a trust fall into the universe. When we are willing to relinquish how we think it all needs to go, we stop being in the way of the most beautiful outcome. We practice setting aside our desire for a particular outcome, our perceived need for security or reassurance, and even our opinions about the people we encounter, and suddenly the day feels much more like a grand adventure.

ON THIS BRIGHT DAY,
I WILL SET ASIDE WHAT I THOUGHT I KNEW,
WHAT I THOUGHT I WANTED,
AND BE OPEN TO A NEW EXPERIENCE.

BLE MOVEMENT

Most leaders are indispensable,
but to produce a major social change,
many ordinary people must also be involved.
— ANNE FIROR SCOTT

BLE is a growing worldwide movement of sustainable weight loss and recovery from food addiction. It is a fellowship of people who have acknowledged that the processed foods that comprise most of what people eat today warp our brains and hijack our ability to make empowered choices. As the reality of that truth spreads around the world, we become walking billboards signaling to others what is possible when you adopt a structured way of eating. We are shining testimonials that Bright Lines produce freedom and that nourishing our bodies with food that feels aligned and supportive of our life force is a powerful way to live. You do not have to do a thing to further the movement; you are already a part of it. Just show up as your beautiful self and be a walking testimony that life without sugar and flour is not only possible but joyous.

ON THIS BRIGHT DAY,

I WELCOME MY ROLE IN SPREADING
THE BRIGHT LINE EATING MOVEMENT
AROUND THE WORLD.

July

July 1

UNSTOPPABLE

I can accept failure.
Everyone fails at something.
But I can't accept not trying.
— MICHAEL JORDAN

In Bright Line Eating we do not value perfection. We value being unstoppable. Meaning after a slip, we dig deep and do not diverge from our food plan when we are really tempted. Meaning we reach out and make phone calls when we do not want to. We meditate when it feels uncomfortable and we do our evening habit stack when we are tired. We bookend social engagements. We skip situations that may present overwhelming temptations. We choose our food sobriety over and over again.

When our habits start to wane and our support dwindles, it is time to return to the basics and increase our commitment to this simple program. Being unstoppable means we have an abiding commitment to lead the healthiest life we can live. The only way to fail is to stop trying.

ON THIS BRIGHT DAY,
I RECOMMIT TO SOME PART OF THE BLE PROGRAM
THAT HAS ELUDED ME.

FOOD THOUGHTS

I can resist everything except temptation.
— OSCAR WILDE

We all have food thoughts from time to time. The good news is that there is a world of difference between having a thought about NMF and taking the action to eat it, and in that space lies opportunity. By learning how to turn away from food thoughts, we create the pause to make a choice that supports our recovery.

Feelings often get interpreted as cravings. When we practice interpreting food thoughts not as information about what we want to eat but as insight into an emotion we are having, we change the conversation. If you used to eat every time you felt anxious, when you are anxious during your BLE journey, you may have the thought to eat. But not acting on that gives you access to the actual feelings that underlie your old patterns of coping. Not acting on food thoughts becomes the portal for greater self-awareness and, ultimately, freedom.

ON THIS BRIGHT DAY,

I WILL GET CURIOUS ABOUT THE EMOTIONS THAT
LIE UNDERNEATH MY FOOD THOUGHTS.

July 3
CAFFEINE

There was a tiny range within which coffee was effective, short of which it was useless, and beyond which, fatal.
— ANNIE DILLARD

In recovery we find that people's reaction to caffeine does not always track neatly with their addictive food susceptibility. Some people who are high on the Susceptibility Scale can drink it moderately, while for other people any caffeine can lead to a binge. For this reason, caffeine is not off-limits in BLE, but we advise that you watch your intake carefully and notice how it affects your mood, energy, and cravings.

For years some of us have used sugar and caffeine when our energy was flagging, when instead what we really needed was rest. If you have *any* trouble sleeping, cutting your consumption of caffeine may benefit you. If you find yourself feeling irritable or looking forward to a cup of coffee or tea, notice if you have the same desire now that you are drinking it black. Some of us find that shifting the beverages we drink during our BLE food plan creates more space for a new way of navigating NMF and NMD. In the end, caffeine is not that different from any other substance—if we are honest about its effects, we get clear about the actions to take.

ON THIS BRIGHT DAY,
I WILL NOTICE MY RELATIONSHIP WITH CAFFEINE WITH CURIOSITY.

RESTAURANTS

Integrity, or the lack of it,
touches almost every facet of our lives—
everything we say, every thought and desire.
— NATHAN ELDON TANNER

Many of us weigh and measure faithfully at home but find that in restaurants we indulge in larger portions. The addiction to quantities can linger on long after the addiction to sugar and flour has lifted, and restaurants are a place where quantities can be a problem.

Planning a meal with family or friends, looking at the menu ahead, and weighing—or honestly eyeballing—our portions will ensure that we keep our Lines Bright. But sometimes being spontaneous or impulsive or walking into a restaurant with a deep inner motive to get a sexier, oilier meal is all our inner Saboteur needs to cause us to veer into dangerous territory.

If you find yourself suggesting dinner out at the last minute, get curious about your motives. Are you "bored" with your simple BLE food? The minute we look for excitement in our food versus in our life, we are on a slippery slope for the addiction to kick up again.

ON THIS BRIGHT DAY,
I AM CAUTIOUS ABOUT RESTAURANTS
AND WILL GET EXTRA SUPPORT IF
I WILL BE EATING OUT.

July 5

SURROUND YOURSELF WITH SUPPORT

Snowflakes, leaves, humans, plants,
raindrops, stars, molecules, microscopic entities
all come in communities.
The singular cannot in reality exist.
— PAULA GUNN ALLEN

With thousands of food cues throughout our environment and the potential for hundreds of food decisions each day, we can be pulled in many directions and get so willpower-depleted that our oldest neural pathways kick in and we break our Lines.

Having supportive people who do BLE and are part of our daily network of conversation will help normalize what some perceive as an extreme lifestyle. If you have multiple prongs of support all around you throughout the day, you will take the BLE way of eating as the norm, which helps it become automatic and deeply ingrained. For some, daily connection through the online community is enough. Others need multiple phone calls. Also be mindful that if you have introverted tendencies you need to be particularly honest with yourself about the distinction between healthy alone time and unhealthy isolation. Immerse yourself in support and notice how Bright your Lines become.

ON THIS BRIGHT DAY,

I WELCOME MY PLACE IN THE BLE COMMUNITY.

P.M. RITUAL

A ruffled mind makes a restless pillow.
— CHARLOTTE BRONTÉ

A Bright Day is actually born at sunset the night before. Having an evening habit stack can help you wind down the day without excess food, which many of us once relied on to get to sleep. It also helps prepare us for the next day, ensuring a Bright Line success.

Some evening rituals include wiping and shutting down the kitchen for the day, writing down our food and committing it to someone, reviewing our calendar of appointments for tomorrow, lowering the lights early to ensure seven to eight hours of sleep, taking a hot bath, doing some yoga or gentle stretching, turning off all screens by a certain time, writing in a five-year or gratitude journal, or reading something uplifting. Taking the time to reflect on our day and notice if we were tempted to eat off plan—and note what allowed us to keep our Lines Bright—can help us prepare for success tomorrow.

Truly, the day begins at sunset the night before.

ON THIS BRIGHT DAY,
I WILL DO MY NIGHTTIME ROUTINE AND
HAVE A PEACEFUL MIND BEFORE BED.

PARTIES

People rarely succeed unless they have
fun in what they are doing.
— DALE CARNEGIE

Before living Bright, parties may have been one big excuse to eat and drink to excess. In fact, looking forward to what was going to be served may have overshadowed looking forward to the opportunities for connection or the event itself. Wonderfully, when the potential to graze on NMF and NMD is removed, over-indulging stops being the focus and other benefits emerge. We can seek out those we are eager to see, make new friends, or ask someone who is off by themselves: "What is new in your world?" or "What has got your attention these days?" These are forms of service that get us out of ourselves and actually become the gateway to a truly good time.

To set ourselves up for success at parties, we must plan ahead. If we want to eat at a party, we might call in advance and find out what is going to be served. If there won't be any vegetables, we might want to bring our own. Sometimes we will choose to eat before or after, which might feel disappointing at first, but we soon find that the removal of that distraction will enable better connections with friends and family than we have ever known.

ON THIS BRIGHT DAY,

I EMBRACE SOCIAL GATHERINGS FOR THE CHANCE
TO BE WITH FRIENDS AND MEET NEW PEOPLE.

FOCUS ON PEOPLE

> I think, at a child's birth, if a mother could ask
> a fairy godmother to endow it with the most
> useful gift, that gift should be curiosity.
>
> — ELEANOR ROOSEVELT

When our food is firmly Bright, we have the mental space and emotional capacity to focus on others. If you are someone who always took care of others and made their lives more important than your own, you may have used food to compensate for that imbalance. Now your focus can shift to the capabilities of others and how they can solve the issues in their own lives while you give yourself the care you had previously denied.

If, on the other hand, addiction left you pretty self-absorbed, then Bright Line Eating will open a vista of opportunity to consciously think about the people in your life and how you can connect with them, support them, and make their lives better. Tune into someone else, let them share their story, and expand your empathy for others.

ON THIS BRIGHT DAY,
I THINK OF BEING OF SERVICE AND REMEMBER
TO BRING BALANCE TO MY LIFE.

July 9

CURIOSITY OVER JUDGMENT

Those who would know the world,
seek first within their being's depths.
— RUDOLF STEINER

If we break our Lines, the invitation is always to approach the situation with curiosity rather than judgment. Shaming ourselves just adds proverbial fuel to the fire of addiction, whereas choosing compassion for ourselves and getting curious about *why* the break happened allows us to notice something new about our motives, triggers, and reactions.

This is a learning opportunity. How can you do something differently moving forward so you do not find yourself here again? Does some part of you have resistance to the program? Do you have too much on your plate? Did you put yourself in a challenging situation too early in your program without enough support? Be a scientist and collect the data so you can make different choices moving forward.

ON THIS BRIGHT DAY,
I WILL APPROACH THE WORLD, MY INNER LIFE,
AND MY BLE PROGRAM WITH CURIOSITY.

FREQUENCY OF CONNECTION

The first duty of love is to listen.
— PAUL TILLICH

There is something to be said for solitude and keeping a small circle of intimates, but sometimes it can unintentionally blur into isolation. While introverts prefer fewer friends but deeper connections, extroverts get lit up by a variety of connections, and even superficial interactions with strangers can be a big boost.

It is important to take stock of how much connection we need and how deeply we want to talk with other people. These are important pieces of self-knowledge. Through that lens, how often are you in contact with another Bright Lifer? How often do you contact your oldest friends? Do you regularly connect with extended family? Neighbors? Take the time with colleagues to learn how they really are?

The way to build lasting, meaningful friendships with others in BLE is to have some regular contact rather than random phone calls. Consistency, frequency, and intimacy all factor into the depth of relationships, and in the end, that is what will help you stick to your Bright Lines in any circumstance.

ON THIS BRIGHT DAY,

I WILL REACH OUT TO SOMEONE I HAVE NOT
CONNECTED WITH IN A WHILE.

July 11

THERE IS ALWAYS HOPE

We must accept finite disappointment,
but we must never lose infinite hope.
— MARTIN LUTHER KING JR.

We have a saying in recovery, "No matter how long you have been on the road, you are always still two feet from the ditch. And no matter how long you have been in the ditch, you are always still just two feet from the road."

If you are in the ditch, you may feel hopeless. Sugar and flour can make our thinking desperate and negative. The good news is that if you have been off your Bright Lines, it does not take long eating squeaky clean to feel hope again. Talking to someone working a strong BLE program becomes a pathway to that hope. We know you can do this long before you believe it. Take the actions that a hopeful person would take, watch your feelings change as you do these actions, and notice what beliefs begin to form because everything is now slightly different.

If you have no hope that you, too, can keep Bright Lines every single day, talk to someone who does, ask them what actions they take, and apprentice yourself to their program. Chances are what they say will inspire you to do the same, even if just for today.

ON THIS BRIGHT DAY,
I SUMMON HOPE FOR MY PROGRAM.

July 12
ENERGY AUDIT

Life engenders life. Energy creates energy.
It is by spending oneself that one becomes rich.
— SARAH BERNHARDT

Before recovery we may have used sugar or caffeine to get a quick hit of energy. Now we have to be more in tune with how we spend and bolster our energy. Gossip and criticism are drainers of energy as are situations involving a lot of conflict and elements over which we have no control. Getting sucked into the news or political turmoil over which we do not have any control can also be depleting.

Where are you leaking energy? Where is your energy out of balance? Do you need to sleep more? Have more support? What will you do differently now to expend bottled-up energy? Will you be of service, create something, or move your body?

What will you do differently today to increase your energy? Build in a break? Go to bed earlier? Dance in the kitchen to some music? Be more conscious of your breath? Call a friend?

What brings you subtle energy every day? Playing with animals? Spending time with children? Reading a good book or taking a walk in nature?

When we realize we have the power to avoid many of our energy drainers, and the power to practice many of our energy boosters, we have more to give our program and our life.

ON THIS BRIGHT DAY,

I WILL BE A WISE STEWARD OF MY ENERGY.

BELONGING

No written law has ever been more binding than
unwritten custom supported by popular opinion.
— CARRIE CHAPMAN CATT

Becoming a Bright Lifer is about more than just being one of
many people who eat the way you do. It is about belonging to
a community of people willing to do something difficult, even
countercultural; it is about adopting a new identity.

Belonging does not happen overnight and does not occur
only by invitation. We are going to feel like we belong if we have
taken actions to show ourselves that we are part of this community, which is often made up of people who felt like they did not
belong in other places. Our feeling of belonging is in our hands.
Belonging brings with it the responsibility for the health of the
community, a commitment to act from our Authentic Self, and
a generosity of interpretation when someone hurts our feelings.
If BLE is where you want to belong, we welcome you right now!

ON THIS BRIGHT DAY,
I SURROUND MYSELF WITH PEOPLE
WHOSE THINKING, ACTIONS, AND IDENTITIES
AROUND FOOD SUPPORT ME.

REBEL ENERGY

Better to die fighting for freedom than be
a prisoner all the days of your life.
— BOB MARLEY

Some of us used food to rebel against demands, responsibilities, and obligations that we were not capable of saying no to, for whatever reason. That may leave us with a Rebel part that sees Bright Line Eating as restrictive. If we find that we have a strong Rebel part of us that is sabotaging our success, then part of us might need help understanding that we are *choosing* Bright Line Eating and no one is forcing it on us.

That Rebel part can also be redirected and redeployed to fight against, for example, the food industry that is spending billions to keep us hooked and buying their products, regardless of the negative health and societal consequences. Learning who your inner Rebel is, what they really want, and where they might be helpful in your life becomes an interesting process once your Lines are Bright and you can notice the first moments of Rebel energy.

ON THIS BRIGHT DAY,

I USE THE REBEL INSIDE ME TO FIGHT FOR
MY LIBERATION FROM NMF.

July 15
ACKNOWLEDGING PROGRESS

Coming together is a beginning;
keeping together is progress;
working together is success.
— EDWARD EVERETT HALE

We often focus on the gap between where we are now and where we ideally would like to be, especially when it comes to our weight. It takes effort to intentionally focus on how far we have traveled, but we will do well to spend that effort, for redirecting our focus away from dissatisfaction and onto all the progress we have made will make for a far more joyous and contented journey.

If you only define success as arriving at your goal weight, you'll miss all kinds of opportunities along the way to celebrate keeping your Lines Bright, including the milestones of weight loss and the development of your character. So rather than noting where you aren't, what size you are not wearing, or how far you have yet to go, pay attention to the subtle, steady changes and shifts that come from living within the Bright Lines. You will find a daily source of contentment that adds to your hope and contributes to your momentum. Falling in love with your personal growth means noticing the progress in all areas of your life.

ON THIS BRIGHT DAY,
I TAKE NOTE OF THE PROGRESS I HAVE MADE
IN AREAS THAT MATTER TO ME.

KNOW YOUR HISTORY

Armed with the knowledge of our past,
we can with confidence charter a course for our future.

— MALCOLM X

Our history can be a goldmine of insight and information for how to chart a course moving forward. Part of creating a strong program of recovery from food addiction is knowing what patterns, situations, and thoughts have derailed us in the past. Knowing our history and being honest about it becomes a foundation from which we launch the next chapter.

It is important not to let our addictive brains minimize the pain we experienced or caused. In BLE, we do not dwell in the past or shame ourselves for old behaviors. Instead, we learn from them, welcome the growth, and invite our Authentic Self to show us a different way. The BLE program has so many tools that help us create new neural pathways, including reaching out when we are struggling *and* when life is good. Understanding when you tend to isolate and what old stories occupy your mind will be a powerful step toward taking a new way, one that leads to freedom.

ON THIS BRIGHT DAY,

I WILL EMBRACE MY HISTORY AS A
TREASURE TROVE OF INSIGHT.

July 17
COMPLACENCY

Be a yardstick of quality. Some people aren't used to an
environment where excellence is expected.
— STEVE JOBS

One definition of insanity is to find something that works and stop doing it. Oftentimes when we get to our Bright Body, we let up on the very actions that helped get us there. Maybe we stop writing down our food because we think we know what we usually eat. Maybe we let our morning and evening habit stacks unravel because we are going through a particularly busy season of life. Maybe we let the program take a back seat because we assume we have automaticity around our four Bright Lines.

Whenever we make the decision to coast, no matter what the reason, it inevitably leads to some kind of slippage in the happiness that comes from living this program wholeheartedly and with complete integrity. It is not always easy to put BLE first, but it is always worth it. Take a moment today to notice if you are coasting—resting on your good work from last month or even yesterday—and commit to being more present and loving with yourself and others as you do exactly what has helped you so far.

ON THIS BRIGHT DAY,
I LEAN TOWARD EXCELLENCE IN EVERY ACTION.

TRUE CELEBRATION

Singing is like a celebration of oxygen.

— BJÖRK

Food has become the center of celebration on religious, secular, and family holidays. This made sense in earlier times when food was scarce and the end of a successful hunt or bounteous harvest culminated in a communal feast. However, nowadays, many celebrations can result in harmful excess eating—and often do.

Because we eat only our three committed meals each day, we sometimes find ourselves at events where others are eating NMF and we are not. One of the gifts we get in this program is the ability to be creative in finding deeper, richer ways to get our fundamental needs met—and that includes learning to celebrate without NMF. Here is the opportunity to truly celebrate at the deepest level of connection with others—to focus on the joy, the accomplishment, and the occasion, or to celebrate the person being honored by giving them our love, attention, and presence. Then we are celebrating the event and celebrating ourself and our commitment at the same time. What joy!

ON THIS BRIGHT DAY,

I WILL CELEBRATE WITH MY FULL HEART.

NO BLE POLICE

You have to be true to yourself,
but you have to be true to your best self,
not to the self that secretly thinks you are
better than other people.

— STEPHEN GASKIN

While there is a clear program that we follow, we also say, "There are no BLE police, and you make your own decisions." We never deny someone their research. The fact is that people are at different places on the Susceptibility Scale and different places in their own journey, so it really is important that we honor everybody's autonomy in crafting their program.

Perhaps you think a certain food or beverage would be okay from time to time in your food plan. See how it works. If you are lower on the Susceptibility Scale, you may have success with it. If you are higher on the Susceptibility Scale, it may or may not work; when you run the experiment, you will find out. For those highest on the Susceptibility Scale, the combined experience of thousands has shown that, on average and in general, *just following the fabulous plan* (JFTFP) is the path that brings about weight loss and peace of mind. But you are not an average, you are a person, so listen to your inner guidance and act accordingly. In the end, do what gives you peace.

ON THIS BRIGHT DAY,

I WILL FOLLOW MY INNER GUIDANCE AND
DO WHAT GIVES ME PEACE.

NEXT STEPS

And the trouble is, if you don't risk anything,
you risk even more.

— ERICA JONG

Because there is no such thing as standing still in life, we have to grow and evolve to take the next step, whatever that looks like. Sometimes the next step is clear—learning about Maintenance and gradually adding food because we are getting down to our goal weight range. But sometimes the next step is subtler and emerges over time as you listen to the signals deep within yourself—picking up your drawing pad again, making amends with an estranged family member, or venturing to a new neighborhood to walk.

Whatever the small nudge is, if you listen and have the courage to act on that guidance, you may find yourself amazed at the synchronicity of events, maybe meeting someone along the way or resting in the quiet contentment of the joy of taking this small risk. Research shows that self-described "lucky" people are simply more open to the nudge of intuition, to taking a risk or trying something new or different in the moment.

Ask yourself today what next steps might be calling.

ON THIS BRIGHT DAY,

I TAKE THE NEXT STEP THAT STRETCHES ME.

July 21

DISCERNMENT

It's exhilarating to be alive in a time of
awakening consciousness; it can also be confusing,
disorienting, and painful.

— ADRIENNE RICH

The BLE life offers more nuanced levels of discernment than were possible when we were in the food. With our food handled, we have the energy to give attention to the rest of life, to the rest of the world, and to our inner state of being. Subtle awareness has time to take root and blossom when our sole focus is no longer on our bodies, our weight, or the endless battle of eating, dieting, resisting, and giving in. We can pay attention to our surroundings and move toward people who truly lift us up and away from people who might be unsupportive. We can hear our inner voice telling us to make career changes or life changes.

Maybe our job is no longer a fit now that we can think clearly and have so much more to give. Maybe we want to be around people and situations that refill our energy instead of depleting it. Learning to listen to the quieter cues also helps inform us if we are not as solidly within the Bright Lines as we would like to be. Heeding those red flags before we are derailed becomes a skillful practice of discernment that opens up greater areas of purpose and joy.

ON THIS BRIGHT DAY,
I WELCOME DISCERNMENT AND TAKE ACTION
ON THE AWARENESS THAT COMES.

July 22
CHAOS

Problems, unfortunately, can be addicting.
Like it or not, we take a certain amount of pride
in the very problems that distress us.
— ELOISE RISTAD

In the throes of addiction, many of us kept our lives unnecessarily chaotic to avoid having to look squarely at our eating. The fender bender made so much worse by lapsed insurance, for example. The more chaos, the better the excuse to comfort ourself with food. Others in BLE may have avoided chaotic situations and relationships because they prized control over everything else, including connection and intimacy.

What is your relationship to chaos, and how has your eating history intertwined with that? Was food your go-to comfort when you experienced calamity in the past or did focusing on food prevent you from entering risky, stretching relationships or activities? Are you using BLE to create another form of chaos today? Slipping and Rezooming all the time can create food chaos in a different form. There is an opportunity in BLE to create a structure of peace using the tools to handle all challenging circumstances. It starts by weighing and measuring the next meal, and welcoming the peace that results.

ON THIS BRIGHT DAY,
I WILL NOTICE IF I FAN MY PROBLEMS INTO CALAMITIES.

July 23
EMPTINESS

If we had a keen vision and feeling of
all ordinary human life, it would be like hearing
the grass grow or the squirrel's heart beat,
and we should die of that roar which lies
on the other side of silence.

— GEORGE ELIOT

Most of us fear emptiness. We ate whenever the first twinge of hunger occurred, filled our car with sound the minute we got in, crammed our calendars with too much to do. The BLE path requires some emptiness, but we also have an opportunity to make friends with it. Perhaps it is the space between three meals, when we actually process all our food thoroughly and even get a little hungry before eating again. Perhaps it is carving time in the day to meditate and sit without an agenda for 10 minutes. Perhaps it is the quiet before bed when we reflect on our day and notice what we need to adjust for tomorrow. Eventually, as we come to recognize emptiness and realize it will not kill us, we perceive it as spaciousness—warm, inviting, and filled with possibilities.

ON THIS BRIGHT DAY,
I LEAN INTO THE QUIET AND THE EMPTY SPACES,
AND LISTEN WITH MY HEART.

July 24

INTEGRITY

The greatness of a man is not in how much
wealth he acquires, but in his integrity and his ability
to affect those around him positively.

— BOB MARLEY

We are now doing what we said we would do, every single day. We are following through on commitments, surprising ourselves with our inner resolve, and offering our full attention, love, and service to others who may be struggling in BLE or other areas of life. We are accomplishing a huge Non-Scale Victory (NSV) with each weighed-and-measured meal by restoring integrity with ourselves.

When the chatter, regret, remorse, or even cheerleading that happened before is quiet, there is an efficiency to integrity that collects your energy into a laser point of focus so that you accomplish more than you thought possible. Bask in this new energy.

ON THIS BRIGHT DAY,

I WILL STRENGTHEN MY INTEGRITY BY WRITING DOWN
MY FOOD AND EATING ONLY AND EXACTLY THAT.

July 25
SHARING

To know even one life has breathed easier because
you have lived—this is to have succeeded.
— RALPH WALDO EMERSON

Giving your support to someone who is struggling feels mar-velous, doesn't it? There is something about sharing kind-ness with someone who is suffering in the precise way that you have suffered that heightens its impact. That form of sharing is special and uniquely effective because we can pass on what has worked for us. It is an honor and a duty.

Passing along practical tips to someone who is about to travel for the first time and helping another navigate the BLE website and find what they need to feel more connected are actions that fill up those inner spaces that food used to occupy. Our shared problem and common solution builds a strong community of support, and it is an ancient truth that giving away what we have allows us to keep it.

ON THIS BRIGHT DAY,
I WILL HELP SOMEONE WHO IS STRUGGLING
WITH A PROBLEM I HAVE EXPERIENCED.

July 26
MEANING

To love what you do and feel that it matters—
how could anything be more fun?
— KATHARINE GRAHAM

Everyone wants to live a life of meaning and purpose. In BLE, when we get our food handled so it is not the be-all and end-all of our lives, we have a chance to create meaning far beyond our body size. Living in a Bright Body is the means to a life of meaning, not an end in and of itself. Stay open to where you are being invited to be of greater purpose and the arenas that call for your unique talents and abilities, and allow yourself to lean into the most meaningful reading, media, and friendships today.

A meaningful life does not have to be grandiose. If each one of us brings love and care and beauty and compassion to those in our immediate surroundings, the world would be a place we would all enjoy living. Each of us just needs to do our part in that and notice the meaning in what we already do.

ON THIS BRIGHT DAY,
I LOOK FOR THE MEANING AND
PURPOSE IN WHAT I DO.

CROSSROADS

There are two ways to go when you hit that crossroads
in your life: There is the bad way, when you
sort of give up, and then there is the really hard way,
when you fight back. I went the hard way
and came out of it okay.

— MATTHEW PERRY

Sometimes we are aware that we are standing at a crossroads, a point in life where we have to make a definite decision and walk along a new path. Coming into BLE is that crossroads for some of us, and we have never looked back. Others find themselves facing a crossroads every single day: Am I going to follow my food plan today or veer off? Making that decision each day, each meal, at every sighting of NMF can be exhausting.

Find a crossroads of identity, make a decision, and move forward with everything you have. That will allow you to face the next, larger crossroads with the best of you leading the way.

ON THIS BRIGHT DAY,

I WILL TAKE THE FORK IN THE ROAD
THAT LEADS TO THE BRIGHT FUTURE
I WANT FOR MYSELF.

July 28

FOOD IS FIRST IN, LAST OUT

Wisdom comes from experience.
Experience is often a result of lack of wisdom.
— TERRY PRATCHETT

We say get the food in order and then build in the habits that create the environment where it is automatic, even easy, to eat Bright. Interestingly, when people slip, food is frequently the last thing to go. Typically, the habits that hold the BLE program in place erode bit by bit, then our identity as a Bright Lifer slips, and at some point, we eat off plan. Keeping the food at the center of our program matters, but so does monitoring how well the habits are holding up. Even though almost all of us do cut a corner on something in our habit stack at some point, the moment you notice you are slipping, make a course correction, buoy it up, and get more support. Your food never has to get wonky if you stay aware of how your habits are holding.

ON THIS BRIGHT DAY,

I WILL PAY ATTENTION TO THE SUBTLE SIGNALS THAT
TELL ME MY LINES ARE ABOUT TO WOBBLE.

LIFELONG LEARNER

Education happens everywhere,
and it happens from the moment a child is born—
and some people say before—
until a person dies.

— SARA LAWRENCE-LIGHTFOOT

If we approach BLE as a diet, once we have studied the food plan and tried it out for a while, we are pretty much done. Of course, our success will not last. The real magic is to fall in love with our journey of personal growth.

We learn about ourselves and about how to grow ever better, ever stronger, and ever wiser on this Bright path. We learn what our trailheads are—those circumstances that trigger us, those places where we feel off track, those old traumas or wounds that suddenly come up and need our care and love.

If we are paying attention, our intuition will tell us where the next chapter of our growth is, and we just have to keep following those signs. If we fall in love with the journey of personal growth, Bright Line Eating never gets old and it never gets dull. There is always more work to do, including learning to be of more service. We never run out of courses in our lifelong learning journey.

ON THIS BRIGHT DAY,
I WILL CELEBRATE THE NEW WAYS
I AM LEARNING AND GROWING.

MONITOR AND ADJUST

If you begin to understand what you are
without trying to change it, then what you
are undergoes a transformation.

— J. KRISHNAMURTI

One of the key pieces of the BLE program is monitoring. We monitor what matters, so the Nightly Checklist is a chance to audit our habits. Which ones do we want to make automatic? Which ones must be done daily in order to keep our Lines Bright? When we find that we have let something slip or we haven't taken an action with our full presence, or perhaps the action has become so automatic that it is time to put another one on the list, then we adjust what we are monitoring. Without a system to monitor, however, the old patterns and pathways can inch their way back into our lives so subtly that we find ourselves eating outside the Lines and have no idea why. Monitoring keeps the basics of BLE front and center in our consciousness.

ON THIS BRIGHT DAY,

I WELCOME ALL INSIGHTS ABOUT MY BEHAVIOR.

July 31
JUST FOR TODAY

If you are caught up in stories about the future,
you are not paying attention to what is happening now.
You are asking for trouble.
— AJAHN BRAHM

The mantra "Just for today" allows us to say no to something we might otherwise want to eat because we are not banning it forever—just for today. And when we are doing something hard voluntarily, "just for today" feels more possible than doing a hard thing for a month—or a lifetime. The part of the brain where addiction lives cannot see that far into the future, is not good with delayed gratification, and cannot even think through the consequences of doing something against our better judgment. So by curtailing the timeline of our commitment to just these 24 hours, we give our brains and bodies a chance to relax into the moment and do what is best.

ON THIS BRIGHT DAY,

I GIVE MYSELF PERMISSION TO WORK THIS
PROGRAM JUST FOR TODAY.

August

August 1
THE SABOTEUR

My fat cells have a memory like Einstein!
I'm proof that surgery is not a magic potion.
There are many ways to sabotage it.

— CARNIE WILSON

Many of us walking this path have years, maybe even decades, of failed weight-loss attempts behind us. When it comes to our food and our weight, we can feel disheartened by the part of us that seems to fight against what we know is in our best interests. The voice that works against our best and Brightest future may be a Food Indulger, a Rebel, or an Isolator, which can operate collectively as the Saboteur.

Each of us has a Saboteur that attempts to derail us from time to time. The challenge with recognizing it is that it speaks in our own voice, so it can sound like inner guidance or common sense. Learning to recognize the seductive, often seemingly rational, suggestions of the Saboteur is a life's work.

Initially, we combat the Saboteur with mantras and strong self-talk, shutting out its perspective and following the original plan, no matter what. Eventually, we come to realize that our Saboteur is a part of us trying to protect us and make us happy and safe—no matter how off-kilter its strategies may be. Our true journey of healing begins with getting curious and finding out what it needs and how it is trying to help.

ON THIS BRIGHT DAY,

I GET CURIOUS ABOUT WHAT MY INNER
SABOTEUR REALLY WANTS AND NEEDS.

PROTECT YOUR CRYSTAL VASE

Life takes on meaning when you become motivated,
set goals, and charge after them in an unstoppable manner.
— LES BROWN

If you have never broken a Bright Line, celebrate and do whatever it takes to maintain your streak. Protect your recovery as if it were a priceless crystal vase. Keep it safe, tend to it, and for goodness' sake, do not juggle with it. Although we can always pick up the pieces and make our program strong again, the gift of not having to do so should not be underestimated. Because when we break once in a blue moon, we set ourselves up for a brain that is hounding us for exceptions. That is not peace.

Sometimes when someone has a long streak of Bright Days, they might grow complacent and think *just one bite won't hurt.* But one bite off plan opens a door to another exception and yet another. And then, because of a psychological principle called intermittent reinforcement, food cravings become incredibly robust and hard to make extinct, and we find ourselves living in a world in which each exception just brings more exceptions. So if you have not made an exception to the food plan, keep going and enjoy the momentum. Nobody ever regretted sticking to their Bright Lines.

ON THIS BRIGHT DAY,

I PROTECT MY BRIGHT LINES AND
CELEBRATE THE PEACE THEY BRING.

PERMISSION TO BE HUMAN

Every great mistake has a halfway moment,
a split second when it can be recalled
and perhaps remedied.
— PEARL S. BUCK

In BLE, we recognize that we cannot always do this program perfectly. At some point, we will slip up on something, whether it is eating NMF, drinking NMD, skipping an action in our morning habit stack, or hurting someone we care about.

Some mistakes really can be remedied right away. Many a small food item in the kitchen has been popped into a Bright Lifer's mouth only to be spit out again immediately and followed up with a quick phone call to a Bright friend to process the near miss. Many a harsh word has been followed by an immediate apology and a commitment to be more kind.

Other mistakes have happened and cannot be pulled back, but they can be learned from, and that is what makes us into extraordinary people over time—the commitment to examination, change, and growth. Each time we miss the mark, we turn to the Permission to Be Human Action Plan (see Resources on page 383)—10 simple but profound questions that invite us to think through what happened, what led up to it, what story we were acting upon, and what action will help move us forward. Through active investigation, every slip is an opportunity to strengthen our program.

ON THIS BRIGHT DAY,
I LET GO OF PERFECTION AND LOOK TO
REMEDY MY MISTAKES MIDSTREAM.

PRECISION ON THE SCALE

Virtues are formed in man by his doing the actions.
— ARISTOTLE

Food addiction is not just a substance addiction; it is a process addiction. Like gambling or shopping, for some of us the behavior of eating itself has become addictive. And that is why we need boundaries around it.

Precision on the scale gives us a very clear boundary. When we cross it, it is the equivalent of the first sip for an alcoholic. Being precise when you weigh your food frees your brain to stop keeping score and compensating for anything over or under exact quantities. Precision with our food is what allows us immense freedom. The saying "The way you do anything is the way you do everything" applies here. When you are committed to weighing and measuring your food, you can abstain perfectly from every bite of food that is not on your food plan. When you know what the "first bite" is and you are 100 percent clear that you are not eating it today, you are completely free.

ON THIS BRIGHT DAY,
I EMBRACE THE PRECISION OF MY FOOD PLAN.

August 5
PUT YOUR PROGRAM FIRST

Objects in motion tend to stay in motion.
Find a way to get started in less than two minutes.
— JAMES CLEAR

Sometimes we are well resourced and full of energy for all the demands of life. Other times we are depleted and hanging on by a thread. It may be all we can do to get through a day with our Lines intact. And that is okay.

In those times it serves us to put our program first. It is the foundation of our self-care and the keystone habit that will help us get back to a well-resourced place quickly. But that does not mean that we have to do everything and do it perfectly. We may have some habits that are anchor habits and therefore non-negotiable, such as writing down our food and completing the Nightly Checklist. But we may have other actions we would like to take but simply cannot manage today, so we lean into our BLE identity by completing our anchor habits and letting the rest go. Every time we move in the direction of our BLE identity, we let our brain (and our Saboteur) know we are unstoppable.

ON THIS BRIGHT DAY,

I WILL PUT MY PROGRAM FIRST AND TRUST THAT
EVERYTHING ELSE WILL FALL INTO PLACE.

August 6
USE TECHNOLOGY

Prior to the Internet, the last technology that had
any real effect on the way people sat down
and talked together was the table.

— CLAY SHIRKY

BLE is a global movement because of technology, and technology enables us to be supported by—and give support to—people all around the world who are walking this journey alongside us. We are reminded we truly are One when we meet people from different cultures who grew up eating different food and yet share our same struggle. We are grateful for the miracle of technology that allows us to know that no matter the time of day or night, there is someone out there in one time zone or another who is here for us.

Notice and be grateful for the global community you belong to. Whether you are someone who has never joined an official online support community or someone who is already totally immersed in that realm, BLE can work wonders for your feeling of belonging in this world.

ON THIS BRIGHT DAY,

I SINK INTO THE MIRACLE OF OUR GLOBALLY
CONNECTED COMMUNITY.

ENTERTAINING

Three grand essentials to happiness in this life
are something to do, something to love,
and something to hope for.

— JOSEPH ADDISON

Most of us thought that entertaining would be difficult with Bright Line Eating, and we felt nervous about hosting a dinner party or large gathering. But what we found instead is that most people are happy to eat our beautiful food. We typically outsource the dessert, NMD, or bread portions of the meal to other guests or simply do not serve them, and the meal is abundant and satisfying. What matters is that we protect our own Bright Lines in our own kitchen. So we often have someone else serve dessert if others are eating it and talk to our guests while that is happening.

If we are hosting a very big party at our house, weighing and measuring our meal first and setting it off to the side can be really helpful. Often we even eat before the guests come, so we can be truly present when they arrive. And anything that we do not eat and would not normally keep in our own kitchen, we pack it up as leftovers and send it home with our guests when they depart. As always, our primary tool is to make it about the people, not about the food. With Bright Line Eating we find that socializing is more fun than ever, and we realize that people have come to connect and be merry, not just to eat.

ON THIS BRIGHT DAY,
I WELCOME PEOPLE WITH A HOSPITABLE HEART.

August 8
WOOP

> If you have something in your life that you'd really
> like to change—or even if you just want to enjoy it even more—
> you'd be well advised to dispense with the trendy "positive
> thinking" approach and give WOOP a try.
> — GABRIELE OETTINGEN

After *The Secret* came out, scientists wondered if you really could just visualize yourself into your dream life. It turned out that the more time people spent visualizing the future, the less likely they were to achieve that outcome.[3] Visualization works to convince our brains we already have attained the goal. It makes our brains relaxed and happy—the exact opposite of the scrappy, risk-taking mindset that leads to, for example, starting a new business and building it up into a thriving success.

WOOP, which stands for Wish, Outcome, Obstacle, and Plan, is a tool we use in BLE to prepare for a challenging situation. It turns out that what really works is visualizing the *obstacles* that might come up between us and our desired outcome and then visualizing how we are going to overcome those obstacles. Being clear on what outcome we want to have (keeping our Lines Bright and not visiting the snack bar in the movie theater, being present for our family by staying off our phones when we play board games, etc.) and then acknowledging what is in the way of achieving that outcome is a great use of our energy.

ON THIS BRIGHT DAY,

I WILL TAKE TIME TO WOOP—TO IMAGINE MY DESIRED FUTURE AND HOW I WILL OVERCOME ANY OBSTACLE.

PUT THE TAPROOT DOWN

Whatever good things we build end up building us.
— JIM ROHN

When times are good and it feels easy to live a Bright Life, that is the best time to anchor your habits. We call it putting the taproot deep into your goodness, into the habits that keep your Lines Bright, and into the relationships that build your support network. Be sure to pick up the phone to celebrate your contentment with other Bright Lifers. Take time to appreciate and savor when a day is going well and write down your gratitudes, the day's highlights, and the good qualities that emerged in you. Good times are when you strengthen those neural pathways and reinforce the positive habits that will hold you steady when the winds of trial and tribulation are blowing fiercely.

ON THIS BRIGHT DAY,

I COMMIT TO PUTTING MY TAPROOT DOWN
AND GROWING MY STORES OF STRENGTH.

August 10
RESISTANCE

What we call ego is simply the mechanism
our mind uses to resist life as it is.

— ADYASHANTI

When we first started this journey, our egoic, addictive self probably protested, "You can't *not* eat sugar and flour *forever*! How will you possibly survive a wedding without wedding cake or your bowling night without pizza?" But we dove in and took it one day at a time.

Resistance comes from inner parts of us that are protecting us. It is the sign of old wounds coming up and impacting us today. And it is the calling card of addiction, so noticing what we are resisting allows us to see how the tendrils of old eating patterns show up, even in our Bright Life today.

The opposite of resistance is acceptance and curiosity. Take a moment to ask, *What am I protecting myself against?* Welcoming resistance as information is the skillful move, because resistance has never gone away by being fought with. What we resist persists, as the saying goes.

ON THIS BRIGHT DAY,

I WILL NOTICE WHERE I MAY BE RESISTING LIFE AS IT IS.

COMMIT TO WHAT YOU CAN CONTROL

I wanted to change the world.
But I have found that the only thing one
can be sure of changing is oneself.
— ALDOUS HUXLEY

Our need for control often shows up in our food journey when we make goals around losing a certain amount of weight by a certain time. We can control putting our food on the scale and having a Bright meal and a Bright Day, but we cannot control how our body does or does not release its weight. Moreover, it is tempting to take score of another's progress or program, to obsess over something that has not happened yet that we think should have, or hyperfocus on what seems to be missing from our life. But we cannot control these things.

Instead, focusing on what is within our control—our actions and our attitudes—is work enough for today (and for a lifetime) for most of us. Rather than giving your energy to trying to control the actions or even the attitudes of those around you, commit to do what you can that is within your control. Make phone calls, plan your meals, and eat what you have committed. These basics deserve your full attention until they are as automatic as brushing your teeth. And then let go of the results and watch your serenity grow.

ON THIS BRIGHT DAY,
I KEEP MY FOCUS ON THE ACTIONS I CAN CONTROL—MINE.

LIVE IN THE SOLUTION

Don't dwell on what went wrong. Instead,
focus on what to do next. Spend your energies on
moving forward toward finding the answer.
— DENIS WAITLEY

Given that we have limited attention, it matters what we give it to—because what we focus on expands. Identifying a problem may be an important starting point on the journey, but dwelling there or talking obsessively about the issue tends to keep our focus on the past.

Turning away from the unpleasant or flawed situation and toward creating the life we do want is what living in the solution means. That is how the promise of the solution expands.

Notice when someone else seems to have an answer, apprentice yourself to that person, and move toward what you truly want, which is not NMF—it is something much grander.

ON THIS BRIGHT DAY,

I WILL KEEP MY FOCUS ON THE SOLUTION
AND WATCH IT EXPAND.

READ THE SIGNS

Through pride we are ever deceiving ourselves.
But deep down below the surface of the average
conscience a still, small voice says to us,
"Something is out of tune."
— CARL JUNG

Every slip begins with a tiny exception. It may be an exception of attitude or it may be one of behavior. For some of us, the signs include a bit more resistance to doing our nightly habits; for others, it is rationalizing a spontaneous meal out or the one-plate rule.

Our Bright Life can be broken down into three categories: food, actions, and support. Generally our actions and our support will slip before the food, so if we can pay attention to our morning and evening habit stacks and to our phone calls and connection in the online support community, we can read the signs that predict that we are headed for a break with our food. One day of missed meditation is generally nothing to worry. But a significant stretch of time where we're sliding lower and lower, where our habits are off track and we're disconnected from our recovery community, could spell trouble. Over time, we learn which signs indicate that we are heading onto the downward slope so we can shore up our support and accountability.

Whatever your subtle signs are, becoming familiar and approaching them with curiosity will allow you to never get low enough on that slope to get into the food again.

ON THIS BRIGHT DAY,
I WATCH FOR SUBTLE SIGNS.

August 14

INNER CRITIC

I'm my own worst critic.
— AMY WINEHOUSE

Many of us have an Inner Critic part who finds something wrong with everything—us, the things we do, the way our loved ones show up, the way the workplace or even the world operates. But listening to this nonstop barrage of criticism can be defeating as we walk a new path of eating and food recovery.

The moment we notice ourselves getting self-critical, comparing ourselves to others, or being unnecessarily judgmental, we remember that this part of us is trying to help. It is looking for acceptance and protecting a part of us that has been hurt from past rejections. Its belief is that if we do everything perfectly, we will be sure to be accepted and loved in this world; its strategy is to berate and browbeat us into perfection.

But that is not the way the world works. People who are tense and critical are not more likely to get love. Our Inner Critic is a little child with simpleminded strategies. It was created as a self-protective mechanism when we were wounded by others as a child, and what it really needs is loving guidance from our own Authentic Self. So we take our Inner Critic by the hand and invite it to experience the liberation of self-acceptance. The more loving we are to ourselves, the more openhearted we feel toward the world—and the more we attract the friendship and acceptance we desire.

ON THIS BRIGHT DAY,
I RELEASE CRITICISM OF MYSELF AND OTHERS.

CHANGE THROUGH LOVE

To love is to make of one's heart a swinging door.
— HOWARD THURMAN

Love powers all lasting change. Sure, we might make a move toward eating better when we are criticized or mocked for our weight, but that cannot be the engine for sustainable change. We shift our identity and change decades-old practices and patterns of consumption because we are loved exactly where we are and invited to be our best selves by those who see that spark in us. Spend time with people who light up when you come into the room, because those people love you and want the best for you.

How do you show yourself love? Following your Bright Lines is one way. How many other ways can you love yourself today for everything you do and all that you are? Sustainable change grows from love, and only you can ignite that within.

ON THIS BRIGHT DAY,
I WILL BEAM LOVE TO MYSELF AND OTHERS.

RATIONALIZATION

Personally, I'm always ready to learn,
although I do not always like being taught.
— WINSTON CHURCHILL

Rationalizing an exception is a tool of our inner Saboteur, that seductive inner Indulger. It is that voice that says, "You deserve that NMF. Just one won't hurt. You have had a hard day, and this will make things better." Or perhaps it asks for increased quantities of BLE foods because, "After all, it's not sugar or flour." That is a tempting rationalization, but one that will slow down weight loss, mess with Maintenance, and enslave us to a lifetime of maddening food chatter.

When we start to hear that part of ourselves negotiate with our food plan or our tools, it is our job to stay firm about why we do what we do. It is a next-level skill to recognize when the inner voice of rationalization and negotiation kicks in and to know right off the bat that it is leading us down an unhelpful path. Because the nature of addiction is that you give it an inch and it takes a mile, and it always hurts, and it is always hard to claw your way back. If you suspect that you are being seduced by your inner Saboteur, use the mantra "None is easier than some—I do *not* negotiate with terrorists!" Or share your food thoughts with someone else in BLE so the food thoughts become externalized and you can hear how unhelpful those ideas actually are.

ON THIS BRIGHT DAY,

I WILL BE AWARE WHEN MY SABOTEUR IS RATIONALIZING.

INNER RESOLVE

Fortitude is the marshal of thought,
the armor of the will, and the fort of reason.
— FRANCIS BACON

Having support is essential to successfully working the BLE program, but even the best network of supportive people, both within and outside BLE, cannot do it all. Walking the BLE path requires inner resolve. Which is different than willpower.

We know that willpower is finite and easily depleted. On the other hand, inner resolve is a deep commitment, renewed daily, to be unstoppable. It is a willingness to do whatever it takes to stick to our food plan, just for today. This inner resolve must be called upon and burnished each morning through prayer, meditation, mantras, and gratitude. And then we take the next right action that signifies that commitment. We demonstrate our inner resolve throughout the day by doing the things that it takes to live a beautiful Bright Day.

Inside of you is a warrior for your Bright self. Allow that warrior to shine.

ON THIS BRIGHT DAY,

I REASSERT MY INNER RESOLVE TO FOLLOW MY LINES.

TRUE DISTRACTION

There never was yet an uninteresting life.
Such a thing is an impossibility. Inside of the dullest
exterior there is a drama, a comedy, and a tragedy.

— MARK TWAIN

It is okay to want to be distracted from life sometimes. So often, food was a handy distraction from a problem, a challenge, or a chore that was not difficult but not pleasant. Food allowed us to focus on something other than feeling socially awkward at a party, and it gave us something to do with our hands during a break at work.

Nobody expects you to be fully present, 100 percent authentic, and doing hard things every moment. But when you let go of mindless eating as an option, it is interesting to notice what provides nourishing distraction. It is usually not something you consume, but rather the act of creating that brings the real relief. Putting your hands in clay, in earth, or on your loved one's tired shoulders can bring real relief from a current trouble. Also, when you bring your attention to creativity, you truly become present.

Notice what is beautiful, savor the moment, and tap into the wonder of how extraordinary it is to be alive.

ON THIS BRIGHT DAY,

I WILL FIND NOURISHING DISTRACTIONS AND
LET MY HEART TOUCH THE SUBLIME.

OVERRELIANCE ON SELF

I say you shall yet find the friend you were looking for.
— WALT WHITMAN

The reason asking for help is so darn hard is that most of us have come to rely on only ourselves for the success of our lives. We learned, often at a very early age, that the adults in our lives were perhaps too busy, or perhaps not emotionally or mentally capable or available, to help us navigate or interpret or soothe. So, we learned to rely on ourselves, developing coping skills based on our strengths that at some point grew maladaptive.

Learning to balance self-reliance with interdependence is an ongoing dance, but as we learn to lean on others, we find a better version of ourselves: one who will ask for help, one who will be vulnerable, and one who will express a want, need, or regret. And the person who is willing to take the risk of being in connection is a more courageous and more admirable version of us than the one who chooses to stay isolated and trudge on alone.

We can fall in love with ourselves all over again by taking the risk of being interdependent. And our recovery will be stronger the more we simultaneously develop the deep skills required to navigate hard times without food and learn to lean on others.

ON THIS BRIGHT DAY,
I WILL TRY RELYING ON OTHERS
MORE THAN I USUALLY DO.

TRUST

Integrity is the essence of everything successful.

— R. BUCKMINSTER FULLER

When we come into recovery, we typically no longer have great trust in ourselves to make the right decisions around food. That is understandable, and probably wise. Trust does not get restored overnight, but BLE is not a program that requires supreme willpower or self-trust; it is a full program that creates an environment that allows our brains to heal and our habits to become as automatic as breathing. You will learn to trust this program if you follow it. If you trust this community with your most vulnerable sharing, trust that this food plan will work for you too, and trust that you should do what is in BLE, you will succeed beyond anything you have imagined.

But trust happens one day at a time, one meal at a time. Integrity starts with the first Bright Day of writing down our food, committing it, and then eating only and exactly that. And when we watch ourselves eat only and exactly that, we have the first glimmers of integrity that become the core of our self-trust. The next day we repeat those actions and allow it to build, one Bright meal at a time.

Restore your self-trust by following through with your commitments and reaching out for support when you do not think you can.

ON THIS BRIGHT DAY,

I RECEIVE THE MIRACLE OF KEEPING
INTEGRITY WITH MY FOOD.

SAYING YES

The only way to say no to anything
is to have a deeper, more important yes.
— MATTHEW KELLY

People who do not understand BLE often think of it as just saying no a lot. No to sugar, no to flour, no to snacking, no to overindulgence during the holidays, and no to letting loose with food and booze on vacation.

But look closer. We are saying yes to a whole lot.

Take the time to get clear on *why* you are doing BLE. You are saying yes to energy, yes to great sleep, yes to playing with the children in your life, yes to better health, yes to joints that do not hurt, and yes to feeling good in your skin. The yeses far outweigh the nos.

Make a mental list of what you are allowing into your life by saying no to sugar and flour. Spend time noticing what is possible when your mind has cleared of food chatter. Lean into what is working, what you truly want, and continue to keep the more subtle traits of serenity, contentment, and equanimity in the foreground. The weight will slip away and NMF will lose its allure when your attention has turned to what you are inviting in.

ON THIS BRIGHT DAY,

I WILL SAY YES!

August 22
HOME

The ache for home lives in all of us,
the safe place where we can go as we are
and not be questioned.
— MAYA ANGELOU

Now that we do not eat to postpone discomfort, we may find ourselves not feeling as "at home" in certain settings or even friendships as we once did. But we now have the opportunity to create a *new* home in routines that serve our body, mind, and soul and that allow us to have the lives we really want and be the people we really want to be. That is a home like no other. And we can access that home within ourselves anywhere in the world.

Finding a sense of home with others who eat the same way we do can also provide a refuge or oasis to negotiate more challenging environments. The BLE community can give us a sense of connection and belonging unlike anything we have ever felt before. Because when we feel at home—in our bodies, our communities, and our corner of the world, we can achieve our potential.

ON THIS BRIGHT DAY,

I KNOW I AM AT HOME WITHIN MYSELF
AND MY COMMUNITY.

LISTENING TO THE SOUL

If I stop chasing what my mind wants,
I will get what my soul needs.
— ANONYMOUS

Learning to listen to what our deepest self knows, wants, and believes takes practice. If the voice of our soul has been drowned out for years by our inner Indulger, that clarity will not appear overnight. None of us knows where the portal to the soul is, but it takes an alignment with how we are eating to get a deeper sense of connection with its calling. We can lean into that deeper truth with curiosity, notice when we are uncomfortable, and recognize that we may need something we have never sought before. Once we have been trusting ourselves to eat what we have committed to eat, we can start trusting ourselves to branch off in our lives and perhaps take risks that we never would have taken before.

What is your soul asking for?

ON THIS BRIGHT DAY,

I WILL STAY STILL AND LISTEN TO THE
QUIET CALLING OF MY SOUL.

August 24
SHAME

Shame is the most powerful, master emotion.
It's the fear that we're not good enough.
— BRENÉ BROWN

Healing from shame is a process. Shame may have interwoven itself into many of our food behaviors, and it does not dissipate overnight, just because we are eating with shiny Bright Lines. But doing the next right thing in BLE will move us toward a healthier, happier sense of ourself so that shame gradually lessens.

Shame melts in the light of shared experience with another, and although our individual details differ, BLE is a community with a common history, a common struggle, and a common path forward. Externalizing your fears, speaking aloud your food thoughts, and noticing the emergence of old behaviors or habits and sharing them with a BLE friend goes a long way toward melting shame. You will discover that you are not alone in your past behaviors or your current struggles, and that is the gift of community in recovery.

ON THIS BRIGHT DAY,
I WILL BE BRAVE ENOUGH TO SHARE MY TRUTH.

CONSISTENCY

Success isn't always about greatness.
It's about consistency. Consistent hard work
leads to success. Greatness will come.
— DWAYNE JOHNSON

There is nothing dramatic, for the most part, about steadily losing small amounts of weight each week until it is time to add a bit more food to maintain a healthy size. It may seem unexciting at times to be taking the same steps toward your goal that you did the day before, and the day before that. But it is the repetition that pays dividends.

Being patient and consistently keeping your Lines Bright is the path to your Bright Transformation. Paying attention to the small moments of happiness or joy along the way will make the achievement of a specific outcome, no matter how miraculous it may seem, something you can take in stride. Hitting your goal weight will not destabilize you if you have been keeping your Lines Bright and consistently making connections in the BLE community. It is another day, and a lovely one at that.

ON THIS BRIGHT DAY,

I TRUST THAT THE BABY STEPS I TAKE TODAY
ARE PART OF A GREAT JOURNEY.

MEDITATION

Meditation is not a way of making your mind quiet.
It is a way of entering into the quiet that is already there—
buried under the 50,000 thoughts the average
person thinks every day.

— DEEPAK CHOPRA

Meditation can take many forms. Its essence is to pause, focus, and breathe so that our attention—which may have been hooked by an old story, a tempting food thought, or a worry about the future—returns to the present moment. Presence is actually what many of us were hoping for when we ate excess food—that hit of dopamine when eating sugar or flour that made everything feel more alive.

Some of us used food to escape the present, and food was a numbing device that allowed us to check out. Meditation invites us into the present moment in the healthiest way possible and creates a practice of noticing instead of freaking out or holding on or controlling. And when we meditate regularly, we build and extend our *pause* muscle, that moment of decision where we can choose to use a tool rather than succumb to an urge. Try meditating for just a few minutes today and every day so that you can receive all the benefits: an increased sense of calm and focus, lowered cortisol, greater happiness, and the improved ability over time to return again and again to the present moment.

ON THIS BRIGHT DAY,

I WILL MEDITATE WITH AN INTENTION TO SETTLE
INTO THE SILENCE AND SAVOR THE TIME.

August 27
HOLDING BACK

Some things cannot be taught,
but they can be awakened in the heart.
— MUHAMMAD ALI

It is tempting to hold back from the BLE program in all kinds of ways. There can be a full holding back, which is not even starting Bright Line Eating when we know we are called to. Many people watch the weekly vlogs for years without ever starting officially. A lot of people do Bright Line Eating halfway, adopting some aspects and not others. Even when we are ostensibly working the program fully, we may find that we are holding back.

Are there various tools or disciplines or recommendations that we are not following? Are we being sloppy with our food? Have we stopped writing down our food? Are we doing it on our own and holding ourselves separate and apart from the community? The reality is that when any amount of addiction is at play, partial efforts often yield abysmal results.

We are likely to get what we want out of this journey if we give it a wholehearted effort. When we dive into the center of our community, do the program wholeheartedly, and reach deeper than we ever have before within ourself, we will see our Lines sparkle and our Bright Transformation take shape.

ON THIS BRIGHT DAY,

I WILL INVENTORY MY PROGRAM TO SEE
WHERE I AM HOLDING BACK.

FEEL BETTER FAST

> There is only one corner of the universe you can be
> certain of improving, and that's your own self.
> — ALDOUS HUXLEY

It is amazing how quickly we feel better once we have put sugar and flour down, given ourselves space between meals, and are eating exactly what we committed in the appropriate amounts. That kind of feeling is well deserved, as so much of our past eating history was a life of misery. It is as if our bodies are letting us know they would *love* to eat in a healthy way, without excess food, and to shed any additional weight we are carrying. Similarly, if we are feeling off, we can reassure ourselves that we are only ever 24 hours away from a day well lived, well committed to, and well executed with all the accompanying good feelings.

When you make an apology that you need to make or shift a relationship in a way it needs to be shifted, or get a really good night's sleep when you are overdue, it is amazing how quickly you feel better. Savor the quick rebound of your sense of ease or optimism, and take it as a confirming sign that being on this journey or getting back on track is exactly the right thing for you.

ON THIS BRIGHT DAY,

I WILL NOTICE WHERE I NEED TO GET BACK
ON TRACK, TAKE A SOLID ACTION, AND CELEBRATE
HOW QUICKLY I FEEL BETTER.

August 29

TAKE MY HAND

I don't know what your destiny will be,
but one thing I do know: the only ones among you
who will be really happy are those who
have sought and found how to serve.

— ALBERT SCHWEITZER

Nobody gets out of the ditch on their own, so there is no shame in asking for help or acknowledging that your Lines are wobblier than you would like and that you need help tightening them up. In BLE, we have so many loving people willing to extend their hand to pull you up when you have fallen. Take the first hand extended to you and come back to the center of the BLE path—quickly, if you can.

If we are solid, then we need to be offering our hand to people who need support. We need to be consciously thinking, *How can I help the person who is still suffering and extend my support to them?* The blessing of having been in the ditch—whether for a moment or for a long time, even repeatedly, even for years or decades—is that when we get Bright again, we have a unique wellspring of experience that allows us to be that much more helpful. Because people who are suffering in that way often need support from someone who understands their pain from personal, lived experience. And if we are the one suffering, we can trust that in time the suffering is going to become our greatest blessing through the fullness of service.

ON THIS BRIGHT DAY,

I OFFER MY HAND TO ANYONE WHO NEEDS SUPPORT.

August 30

BINGEING

Privation is the source of appetite.
— SOR JUANA INÉS DE LA CRUZ

Some people come to BLE with a history of binge eating disorder. Others have kept themselves going with a steady supply of NMF throughout their days so that once they stop eating sugar and flour, if they slip, they find themselves eating quantities like they never did before.

If you find yourself bingeing, it might be wise to eat the Maintenance Food Plan until your Lines are Bright, and only once your program is truly automatic, gradually reduce to the Weight-Loss Plan. But please know that the part of the brain that says "binge" is not the part in charge of the muscles that pick up the food. No matter what your urges are, those primitive parts of your brain do not control your motor cortex. You always have a choice in how you act.

You are not at the mercy of an inner command to binge. The urge will pass, and if you are able to reach out for help or have a connection you talk to every day, you can share that thought and get support in sticking to your Lines, just for today.

ON THIS BRIGHT DAY,

I WILL NOTICE MY DESIRE FOR MORE FOOD AND
DIG DEEPER TO DISCOVER WHAT I TRULY WANT.

August 31
MAINTENANCE MINDSET

If you were healed of a dreadful wound,
you did not want to keep the bandage.
— URSULA REILLY CURTISS

Maintenance is not radically different from weight loss at all. We still follow our Bright Lines to stay sober. What shifts in Maintenance, then, is the identity of oneself as someone always trying to lose weight.

Now you are someone in a Bright Body who eats to sustain that healthy body. What will you do with all the energy you once devoted to weight loss? What will you do without the hit of joy when the scale goes down? Can you transfer that joy to the satisfaction of maintaining—of staying within your goal range? Or even better, can you listen to what your larger purpose in life might be and find joy, pursuit, and motivation there?

When we move beyond thinking about the food and the weight, we get to hear the calling of our bigger purpose. For many of us, a huge amount of our life focus was devoted to the problem of food and weight, and once that has resolved, we get to reallocate those resources to more worthy, inspiring, and gratifying pursuits.

ON THIS BRIGHT DAY,
I MOVE PAST THE FOOD AND THE WEIGHT
TO LISTEN TO MY CALLING.

September

September 1
FOOD AS FUEL

I am building a fire, and every day I train, I add more fuel.
At just the right moment, I light the match.
— MIA HAMM

There is one thing that food does best for us, and that is fuel our body and brain. But thinking of your meal as fuel can be a radical departure for those of us who conceived of food as a best friend, a comforter, and the chief source of entertainment. Truly, food is a poor proxy for all those things. As we recover, we find better ways to meet our deeper needs through practice, experimentation, and allowing others in food recovery to guide us to a new way of living.

Of course, we do get pleasure from food and there is nothing wrong with that. We can revel in the pleasure of eating our Bright meals and celebrate that we get to do it three times a day. But to take food out of those other categories and put it into the category of fuel means enjoying eating healthy and wholesome food without looking for it to fulfill unnecessary roles.

ON THIS BRIGHT DAY,

I WILL BRING AWARENESS TO THE ROLE FOOD FILLS IN MY LIFE.

September 2

REZOOM WITH SPEED

*One can never consent to creep when one
feels an impulse to soar.*

— HELEN KELLER

Breaks are always valuable if we seek the lesson and make changes in our program to ensure that we do not fall for the same vulnerabilities in the future. Did we have a lapse in our self-care rituals, cut corners on our healthy habit stacks, skip out on our social support? Did we put ourselves in a situation too tempting or too stressful too early in our recovery journey?

If you break your Bright Lines, Rezoom as quickly as possible. Do not fall for the "what the hell" effect and eat everything you can because you will "just start over tomorrow." That diet mentality is not helpful with your emerging identity as a Bright Lifer. Quickly come back to your weighed BLE foods at your next meal with great self-compassion.

We come from a background of "all or nothing" thinking, but getting back on track and being Bright for the remainder of the day is a huge win and new behavior for so many of us. That in and of itself is worth celebrating.

ON THIS BRIGHT DAY,

I NOTICE WHEN I AM VEERING OFF TRACK AND
COURSE-CORRECT QUICKLY.

FINISH-LINE ANXIETY

When things go badly, it is your fault, not theirs.
You are responsible. Analyze how it happened,
make the necessary fixes, and move on.

— COLIN POWELL

No one in Bright Line Eating is going to tell us what our goal weight range should be—we get to choose—and there is no magic formula telling us what we should weigh. But if you are chronically hovering above where you truly want to be, that resistance could be fear of what else you might need to address in your life if you no longer have the distraction of the food and the weight to focus on. Invite that resistance, fear, or old story to come forth to be addressed.

Are you someone who gets close to your goal but stops short? Are you eating enough BLTs to prevent landing in your goal range? Perhaps it is time to journal about what it would look like to be in your Bright Body? What work would be finished? What work would just be beginning? What possibilities for your life can you glimpse but perhaps do not feel ready for? On the other side of that exploration is the freedom and peace you have been craving.

ON THIS BRIGHT DAY,

I WILL RELEASE OLD FAILURES AND FOCUS ON WHAT IS NEXT.

NEXT BRIGHT MEAL

The next message you need is always right where you are.

— RAM DASS

Focusing on the long term is not helpful during weight loss because leaving behind some of our favorite foods, hangouts, and eating behaviors may feel impossible to do forever. Which is why we reinforce the mentality that there is no forever; there is just this next moment, and then the next one.

When you find yourself overwhelmed with the work of the BLE program, return your focus to the present moment and make preparations for your next Bright meal. That is all you ever have to focus on to be successful here. That is how people string together days, months, and eventually years and decades of shiny Bright Lines. One Bright moment at a time.

ON THIS BRIGHT DAY,

I TRUST THAT THE REST OF MY LIFE WILL WORK OUT
IF I JUST TAKE CARE OF MY NEXT BRIGHT MEAL.

NIGHTLY CHECKLIST REVISITED

Part of having a strong sense of self is to be accountable
for one's actions. No matter how much we explore motives
or lack of motives, we are what we do.
— JANET GERINGER WOITITZ

It is a great irony that the very thing that lets us know our BLE program is slipping is sometimes the first thing to go. Without a checklist each night to review the habits we actually performed that day to keep our BLE program strong, we may convince ourselves all is well, when in fact, we are nearing a danger zone.

BLE is a whole program, inviting many points of connection and many actions that replenish willpower, in addition to the four Bright Lines. Learning how many tools you need to use to keep your Lines Bright is the most important point of this reflection. You are doing it for you, not for anyone else. Noticing that your happiness is lower on days you do not talk to another Bright Lifer matters. Noticing that your cravings are stronger on days you did not get seven to eight hours of sleep can help you make an adjustment. You are a unique person, in a state of growth and change, so keep your Nightly Checklist accurate, up to date, and stay current with your BLE program for maximum success.

ON THIS BRIGHT DAY,

I REVISIT MY NIGHTLY CHECKLIST TO SEE IF IT REFLECTS
WHAT I NEED TO DO TO KEEP MY LINES BRIGHT.

September 6
NEUROPLASTICITY

The chief function of the body is to carry the brain around.
— THOMAS A. EDISON

In recovery we are creating the asset of a brain that functions in a way that will support our most peaceful, vibrant, and flourishing life far into the future. We are lucky that at all ages our brains can heal and rewire. That is why BLE is based on brain science.

Making new neural pathways is hard at first for adults, like hacking through a forest with a machete. However, the more you walk the path, the easier it gets. If our cravings are not as strong as they once were, that is because our dopamine receptors have replenished. If we are feeling just a bit more satisfied at the end of meals, that is because our brain is now able to see more of the leptin that is circulating in our blood and because the inflammation has gone down in the hypothalamus. If weighing and measuring our food is easier than it used to be, that is because fiber tracts are formed in the brain to support those habits. What we do today will inch us ever closer to having a brain that will support doing this with ease long into the future.

ON THIS BRIGHT DAY,
I BRAVELY AND BOLDLY MAKE NEW CONNECTIONS.

September 7

LETTER TO YOUR FUTURE SELF

Danger, Will Robinson!
— *LOST IN SPACE*

If we have been in the ditch recently, off our Lines, eating off plan, and unhappy about it, we can use that information to write a letter to our future self who might consider jumping off plan. Remind them of the physical and emotional experience of feeling out of control with the food again. Alert them to the warning signs that a relapse is coming and remind them they can Rezoom at any time.

This letter of loving advice can be stored somewhere safe, on our phone, or in plain view. The point is to use the experience to learn, grow, and change so it never has to happen again.

ON THIS BRIGHT DAY,
MY HARD-WON BRIGHT GAINS ARE A LOVING
SHIELD AGAINST FUTURE BREAKS.

September 8
OKAY BEING OKAY

Happiness is when what you think, what you say,
and what you do are in harmony.
— MAHATMA GANDHI

For those of us with brains that are more susceptible to addiction than average, we may find that we have gotten used to a certain amount of chaos or swirl in our lives. There may be parts of us that are really attached to the story of what is wrong in our lives. As we recover, we may find that there are lulls when, frankly, we are fine. There is no drama. There is nothing major going on. And we may find it very disconcerting. There is still a part of us that is scanning for *What's wrong? What's my issue? What's my drama?* It may be unsettling to not have that radar land on anything in particular.

This is the time to learn how to be okay. To be able to say to our friends on our food recovery journey, "You know what? I think I am doing fine. There isn't anything to discuss. I am really grateful." There is going to be a learning curve; be patient. Okay you is a new you, and you might need time to grow into it. Start today.

ON THIS BRIGHT DAY,

I CAN LOOK FOR A MOMENT WHEN ALL IS WELL
AND PRACTICE BEING OKAY.

WHAT IS YOUR *WHY*?

There is something in every [person] that waits [and] listens for
the sound of the genuine in [herself] . . .
— HOWARD THURMAN

Knowing why we are doing all the work for BLE matters, especially as we get into Maintenance and weight loss is no longer
the main driver. When we are our best selves, the ones not giving
over any more of our mental real estate to the trivialities of what
we have eaten or not eaten, we can hear the deepest calling and
be freed up to follow our best, Brightest path.

While most people join BLE to lose weight, get healthier, and
feel more at home in their bodies, knowing what you want to do
in that healthier Bright Body will at some point become clearer.
What is the calling of your soul? It could pertain to family,
career, or even healing trauma. When you find yourself debating whether or not to stick with the program today, review your
reasons for eating this way and deepen the *why* of your program.

ON THIS BRIGHT DAY,

I WILL LISTEN TO WHY I WANT TO FOLLOW THE BLE PATH.

September 10

TELLING THE TRUTH

Lying is done with words and also with silence.

— ADRIENNE RICH

Rigorous honesty matters when it comes to gaining traction in this program. For people like us, honesty begins with the food. There are four Bright Lines, and either we are following them or we are not. There may be a temptation to rationalize a bit more of some BLE food or to minimize a one-day break, but being honest about it allows us to ask for the support we need to get back on track. There is no shame in needing help, and nobody expects us to be perfect (except perhaps ourselves). There can, of course, be other aspects of our lives that we are not being honest about that go well beyond the food. But we start with the food, then look at our habits, then look at our support connections, and then circle out from there, taking inventory.

What are we keeping even from ourselves that needs to be revealed? Telling the truth requires great courage and vulnerability, but it is rewarded with the gift of more integrity, more happiness, and more authentic relationships.

ON THIS BRIGHT DAY,

I WILL FIND THE TRUTHS I MAY HAVE BEEN HOLDING BACK, EVEN FROM MYSELF.

TWO FEET FROM THE DITCH, TWO FEET FROM THE ROAD

Commitment is an act, not a word.

— JEAN-PAUL SARTRE

The truth of this recovery journey is that no matter how long you have been walking down this road, you are always still just two feet from the ditch. Which speaks to the need to maintain vigilance—even over the long haul. Do not take your stride for granted. Each step on the road is a gift and every Bright Day is an accomplishment.

Any BLT or NMF or NMD could trip us into the ditch. The ditch is always there. But joyously, the inverse is also true. No matter how long you have been in the ditch, you are still just two feet from the road. It is not a long way back, but it will require help and support and telling the truth. Those walking the road are here for you. Find someone whose program you admire and ask for their support. Talk to them daily until you, too, have a solid and shiny program again.

ON THIS BRIGHT DAY,

I TAKE NO STEP OF MY JOURNEY FOR GRANTED.

DISPLACE YOURSELF

It's a good thing to have all the props pulled out
from under us occasionally. It gives us some sense of what
is rock under our feet, and what is sand.

— MADELEINE L'ENGLE

Living within a comfort zone can feel safe and, well, comfortable. However, it is easy to grow complacent with the same routine, the same food, the same path to work, and the same circle of like-minded people. Rapid growth happens when life displaces us and we are suddenly up against our prejudices, our old coping mechanisms, and our fears.

Research on self-described "lucky" people shows that one of the things they do differently is sprinkle novelty into their day. They are more likely to take a different route to work, try something they have never tried before, and embrace variety.[4] So rather than waiting for life to displace you with a tragedy, try stretching yourself by choice. Give yourself the gift of doing something differently. It could be as simple as journaling in a different location or as big as taking a trip to somewhere you have never been. Know this is a beautiful period of growth and let your circle of support allow you to brave your *dis*comfort zone.

ON THIS BRIGHT DAY,

I INVITE SOMETHING DIFFERENT TO HELP WAKE ME UP.

SELF-CARE BEFORE OTHERS

I had to succeed. I would never stop trying, never.
A violinist had his violin, a painter her palette.
All I had was myself. I was the instrument that I must care for.

— JOSEPHINE BAKER

That maxim from the airlines, "Put on your own oxygen mask before you help someone else," applies in the areas of self-care during recovery as well. If your cup is not filled up, with your willpower replenished and your Lines Bright and shiny, you may not have enough to offer to those you love.

So many of us have been socialized to put the needs of others before our own and have interpreted self-care as being selfish. In truth, as adults, it is nobody's job but our own to take care of ourselves. Food may historically have served as compensation when we were not taking true care of our body by resting, moving, or playing. Now it is our job to discover how to care for ourselves through healthy choices, Bright meals, and reviving relaxation. We have amazing gifts to give in this world, and it is a privilege to take care of ourselves so that we can show up fully.

ON THIS BRIGHT DAY,

I WILL TAKE EXQUISITE CARE OF MYSELF SO I CAN
BE OF MAXIMUM SERVICE TO OTHERS.

September 14
INDULGER ENERGY

When people are wrapped up in themselves,
they make a pretty small package.
—ATTRIBUTED TO HARRY EMERSON FOSDICK

All of us who overate have an inner Food Indulger who tells us all kinds of stories: that just one piece of NMF won't really hurt, that we can start again tomorrow, and that we can control our binges this time. This voice has been active for years and needs to be heard and loved—but not heeded. Feeling deprived is not a sustainable path in recovery. Can you give your inner Indulger something else to indulge in? Does the Indulger want a long bath, a nap, or a phone call with your best friend? Make a list of what you consider real indulgences and notice if you can give yourself permission to do those regularly. Not every indulgence requires money or involves food.

ON THIS BRIGHT DAY,

I NOTE WHAT I TRULY WANT AND GIVE MY INNER
INDULGER SOME LOVE AND ATTENTION, WITHOUT FOOD.

NO ADVICE, JUST PRESENCE

Please give me some good advice in your next letter.
I promise not to follow it.
— EDNA ST. VINCENT MILLAY

If you are working with someone who is struggling, the best thing you can do is listen. When someone is trying to get back on track, it is typically not more information they need but something more nuanced and subtle: the companionship of someone who believes they can do it even when they do not know it themselves.

This is true for anyone in our life going through something hard—our kids, our life partner, our aging parents, our co-workers. So many of us are trying to control and manage others. What a gift it is when we take that energy out of the equation and replace it with peace and openhearted acceptance. If they are also in recovery, they will find their way eventually, and just being with them while they come back is immensely gratifying. Refrain from giving advice or engaging their inner Rebel. You do not need to take on the role of their Food Controller, just be loving and kind with them and watch them bloom.

ON THIS BRIGHT DAY,
I WILL SHOW UP WITH UNCONDITIONAL,
LOVING ACCEPTANCE.

September 16
WOBBLY LINES

The more constraints one imposes,
the more one frees one's self.
— IGOR STRAVINSKY

Wobbly Lines are a sign that it is time to get more support, up your intention and commitment level, and become more precise. Wobbly Lines typically precede a full break in the Bright Lines, a foray into NMF that may prove challenging to come back from. So take any wobbling in your Lines (not using a scale when at home, eating out more frequently than usual for reasons you can control, switching items because of a whim) as an invitation to look deeper.

If we look closer, we might find a Rebel part that is saying recovery is too strict or a Manager part that is trying to save time by cutting corners. Maybe it is a Seductive Rationalizer or Food Indulger that is trying to get an extra hit off the food. But Bright Lines today will allow us to lean into our calm, clear, Authentic Self. Bright Lines will help us choose the path that leads to the most freedom, the most integrity, and the most self-respect. When we take care with our Bright Lines, we are taking care of ourselves, and it feels amazing.

ON THIS BRIGHT DAY,

I WILL MAKE MY LINES SPARKLE AND NOTICE HOW
MY MOOD AND THOUGHTS CHANGE.

DANGER AND DESTRUCTION ZONE

You don't drown by falling in the water.
You drown by staying in there.
— EDWIN LOUIS COLE

Addiction is defined as a relapsing condition, but relapse is not inevitable. While it is completely human to have emotional ups and downs and to not do all our habits perfectly every single day, there is nothing inevitable about getting into the Danger and Destruction Zone and eating off plan. And we can look to the people who have maintained long, unbroken stretches of beautiful, sparkly, Bright Lines and know that with care and vigilance, we can absolutely stay Bright day after consecutive day.

Adhering to the Lines puts a buffer zone between your emotional highs and lows and this danger zone of using food to cope. Sometimes just slowing down and putting your program first is all it takes. Lean into the actions that restore your willpower and the connections you have that allow you to be supported in your BLE identity and life in general.

ON THIS BRIGHT DAY,
I PAY CLOSE ATTENTION TO MY MOODS, ATTITUDES, AND ACTIONS AND MAKE ANY CORRECTIONS I NEED.

TRUE CONNECTION

*Act as if you might just create something beautiful . . .
authentic and universal. Don't wait for anybody to tell you it's
okay. Take that shimmer and show us our humanity.*

— DANI SHAPIRO

For most of us, how we ate before recovery was a painful secret that we did not reveal to others, which left us isolated in shame. In this community, connecting over our shared struggle lays the framework for a level of vulnerability that we will not often have in other areas of our lives. Some of us find the connections in BLE more authentic and intimate than those with friends we have known most of our lives. That is because BLE requires a high level of honesty, vulnerability, and authenticity to be effective and give the nourishment we need to outgrow our old patterns of eating.

If you are new to BLE, you may find yourself surprised at how open and loving others are in the online community where we never meet face-to-face, and in the many other groups available. Bless your life with the experience of a true connection with another by having the truest connection with yourself that you can.

ON THIS BRIGHT DAY,

I WILL MODEL THE VULNERABILITY AND AUTHENTICITY THAT
IS THE HALLMARK OF OUR BRIGHT CONNECTIONS.

INSANITY

Insanity is repeating the same mistakes
and expecting different results.
— NARCOTICS ANONYMOUS

Insanity is a strong word to describe overeating, but if you look at the statistics, 80,000 people in the United States each year have a limb amputated because of their food choices,[5] and millions of people around the world die each year from forms of heart disease that could be alleviated by a change in diet.[6] We do have an insane food system that subsidizes some of the worst foods for our bodies and offers little by way of support for those farming techniques that are healthiest.

BLE is a sane program, one that requires thought and effort, and brings our life into balance. There may be people who think it is crazy to live without sugar and flour and who panic at the thought of doing so. But if the saying is true that insanity is doing the same thing over and over and expecting different results, we have all run that experiment with NMF and NMD again and again—sometimes for decades. With the data that we have showing what happens every time we pick up these foods, we know that it is insane to live any other way than Bright.

ON THIS BRIGHT DAY,

I MAKE THE SANE CHOICE TO STAY BRIGHT AND ENJOY
THE BALANCE IT BRINGS INTO MY LIFE.

ONGOING SUPPORT

It seemed rather incongruous that in a society
of super sophisticated communication,
we often suffer from a shortage of listeners.

— ERMA BOMBECK

Once we reach Maintenance, it is tempting to cut back on our connections, spend less time in the online community, or drop away from a Mastermind Group or Buddy; but the reality is that we need support to live this way for the rest of our lives.

Research shows that how deeply supported and connected we feel in this world is more closely correlated with health and longevity than the combination of diet and exercise put together. Just as a healthy body of water has an inflow and an outflow, we need to receive, and we need to give. Keeping that support flowing enables us to flourish and reach greater heights, strive for self-actualization, and take on new challenges. It is a profound act when we connect deeply with another human being and when we allow them to connect with us.

ON THIS BRIGHT DAY,

I WILL LISTEN DEEPLY AND SHARE FREELY
WHEN I FIND A KIND LISTENER.

September 21
DISCIPLINE

Freedom is never given; it is won.

— A. PHILIP RANDOLPH

Discipline may have once seemed like a kind of punishment, or something completely unattainable. But the Latin root of the word suggests that we are a *disciple* of our own health and wellness.

Discipline is not willpower or bunching up your will in order to force yourself to do something. What makes discipline possible is automaticity. It is building up a daily structure, little by little, until suddenly the way we live looks like discipline. Also, we are creatures of conformity. Having the identity of a Bright Lifer is going to provide support for the scaffolding of our daily disciplines as well.

When people leave Bright Line Eating, they often find themselves unable to attain the same level of daily discipline that they found within our social structures. To be disciplined is to lean into what is best for ourselves, to establish an environment and rhythm of habits that makes doing the right thing easier than veering off plan. Discipline can be your gateway to freedom.

ON THIS BRIGHT DAY,

I WELCOME THE PROGRAM'S DISCIPLINE AND
NOTICE HOW IT HELPS ME FEEL FREE.

FREEDOM FROM AND FREEDOM TO

We know from painful experience that freedom is never voluntarily given by the oppressor.

— MARTIN LUTHER KING JR.

Inside the restrictions of the Bright Lines, we have so many freedoms to celebrate. Eventually we have freedom from obsessive food thoughts, freedom from thinking about our bodies and our weight, freedom from blood work numbers that portend health challenges, freedom from the oppression of knowing that we are killing ourselves on an installment plan, freedom from bingeing, and freedom from the tyranny of addiction.

We now have the freedom to cross our legs, freedom to buy clothes for events months in advance knowing that they will still fit, freedom to eat peacefully, freedom to enjoy a full range of healthy food, and freedom to choose our next action based on our soul's needs, not our addiction's demands. There is so much to enjoy and be grateful for.

ON THIS BRIGHT DAY,

I WALK AWAY FROM THE OLD WAYS THAT ONCE SOOTHED ME AND INTO A NEW FIELD OF FREEDOM.

SERENITY

One's own self is well hidden from one's own self;
of all mines of treasure,
one's own is the last to be dug up.
— FRIEDRICH NIETZSCHE

A lot of excess eating is done to calm down, take a break, and soothe emotional upset, so learning to find serenity without food will take some practice. Pockets of peace can feel disquieting at first, but as we develop a meditation practice, we will get accustomed to serenity and less used to the inner turmoil that characterized our lives before food sobriety. Noting when we are feeling serene requires astute attention because serenity can often feel simultaneously like emptiness and fullness.

How do you know when you are serene? Conversely, what is an early indicator that you are losing your peace? This level of self-awareness grows as we keep our Lines Bright and pay attention to the inner cues that lead us to eat. Now that we are not acting on them, we can get curious and find out what is really going on. This inquiry will lead us down the path of peace.

ON THIS BRIGHT DAY,
I SUMMON CURIOSITY WHEN FACING THE POCKETS
OF PEACE AND STILLNESS WITHIN.

September 24
SELF-EXPRESSION

The longer you delay saying no,
the bigger the risk that the lid will blow off your
mounting resentment and frustration.

— HARRIET BRAIKER

Learning to advocate for ourselves in an environment that foists NMF on us takes courage. But one of the best things about having boundaries around our food is that it may influence other areas of life, and we may find ourselves having clearer boundaries around relationships and encouraging the same in others. This contributes to the kind of society we want to live in—one that is based in consent, where people respect one another's integrity and share their wants and needs freely, where people do not pressure one another to do what they don't want to do. To contribute our part to a world like that, we need to learn how to hear our "yes" and our "no" deep inside and also learn how to share them.

When you start meeting your own needs, you are less likely to want to please others by abandoning what you truly want. Expressing yourself daily is great practice for navigating the world with newfound confidence and kindness.

ON THIS BRIGHT DAY,

I SHARE MY "YES" AND MY "NO" FREELY WITH OTHERS.

September 25

INTENSITY

When adversity strikes, that's when you have to be the most calm.
Take a step back, stay strong, stay grounded and press on.

— LL COOL J

There is a certain unproductive intensity in the binge, regret, Rezoom cycle, as it often involves a lot of uncomfortable, all-consuming emotion. Staying at the same weight, eating all Bright meals—weighed precisely—three times a day, can seem boring by comparison. But keeping your food boring allows your life to grow Brighter, larger, and more expansive. Instead of using food as the main vehicle for drama and emotion, consider making your food simple and looking for intensity and excitement elsewhere.

Sprinting all out for a minute in an exercise routine can be really healthy. The climax of a movie can get our heart racing. A good tandem jump out of an airplane is the definition of exhilarating. Orgasms are healthy, encouraged, and so very fun. How can you find ways to add more productive intensity into your life?

ON THIS BRIGHT DAY,

I WILL NOTICE WHETHER THE INTENSITY
I ENGAGE IN SERVES ME, AND I WILL
SEEK HEALTHY OUTLETS.

LIFE GOALS

I am luminous with age.
— MERIDEL LE SUEUR

How has your relationship with food affected the goals you have had for your life? Many of us have given too much of ourselves and our time to our addictive relationship with food, and it cost us deeply in many ways. For some, our careers suffered tremendously because the cycle of bingeing and dieting took all our focus. For others, food took the place of healthy relationships or our addiction drove a wedge between us and those closest to us.

Have you found yourself less ambitious, less willing to be vulnerable and intimate with others, or less confident in your talents because of your weight or your patterns of eating? Living Bright unleashes all the incredible potential within you as you navigate the world with new skills, new confidence, and perhaps even new goals. Let yourself dream big because you are developing the skills to accomplish what your heart desires.

ON THIS BRIGHT DAY,

I AM FILLED WITH HOPE FOR FUTURE POSSIBILITIES
I AM ONLY JUST BEGINNING TO IMAGINE.

FOOD COMES FIRST

---

*She had the loaded handbag of someone
who camps out and seldom goes home, or who
imagines life must be full of emergencies.*

— MAVIS GALLANT

Just as we would never leave the house without pants on, we should not leave for the day without our food, packed and ready to go. No matter how hectic our mornings are, prepping our food needs to move into the same nonnegotiable category. If that means we are a little late, we are a little late; but we are not going to leave the house without everything we need for a successful day.

This is especially important when we are traveling or when we are going to eat at a restaurant. To not plan ahead and just expect the environment to offer a BLE-friendly meal at the right time can be risky. Better to prepare our meal the night before and grab it on our way out the door. If there is something available where we are going, terrific. But now we are ready if there isn't, and putting our food first frees our brain for other matters all day long.

ON THIS BRIGHT DAY,

I PREPARE IN ADVANCE AND REJOICE IN THE FREEDOM OF
KNOWING THAT MY FOOD IS SORTED.

September 28
ACCEPTANCE

Everything in life that we really accept undergoes a change.
— KATHERINE MANSFIELD

Accepting what we do not like about our lives may seem paradoxical—shouldn't we resist it? And yet until we accept our situation, body, brain, or family, we will not have any peace, nor the solid foundation to work from if we want change. In other words, allowing what is real to simply be, without judgment or regret, starts a process of appreciating something in the moment and leads to new awareness, which helps us to act differently.

Also, if we think there is something wrong with a person or circumstance in our lives, are we sure about that? Maybe it is exactly the way it is supposed to be to teach us a particular lesson or help us see something in a particular way. Maybe the person we think needs change is exactly where they need to be on their trajectory. Who are we to say that something shouldn't be exactly the way it is right now? It is easier to accept what is working and what feels good, but the real practice comes in tranquil acceptance of everything.

ON THIS BRIGHT DAY,
I WILL FIND ONE THING I HAVE RESISTED
AND ACCEPT IT INSTEAD.

SKIN

I did not just fall in love, I made a parachute jump.
— ZORA NEALE HURSTON

The result of losing weight can be excess skin, which can bring to the forefront our relationship with our bodies. Some people may resist starting Bright Line Eating because they are afraid that they will have a lot of saggy skin at goal weight. But so many people in Bright Line Eating have reclaimed their loose skin and developed such an empowered relationship with it that it becomes one of the best things about their Bright Journey.

We need to normalize excess skin and celebrate it! It is the hallmark of a warrior who has seen the world and is now living in a body that is free and healthy. Learning to love the softness of your loose skin and factoring it into your goal weight are all things that Bright Lifers are good at, so align yourself with those values and love the skin you're in.

ON THIS BRIGHT DAY,
I WILL LOVE EVERY INCH OF MY FAITHFUL BODY.

September 30
TRIGGERS

Suffering does not diminish in intensity
when you make it unconscious.
— ECKHART TOLLE

Triggers are environmental cues that remind us of past experiences, both positive and negative. The addictive brain is highly susceptible to the cues that predict food rewards, so they are going to be potent for us, especially when we first begin recovery. We need to be prepared for them and have a plan for what to do if a situation triggers a craving for NMF or NMD.

Something simple like pause, breathe, and call someone can be enough. But notice that each time we experience being triggered and then do something different than we used to do, we are literally rewiring our brain. We are creating our new life.

Food cues are all around us, and we have the opportunity today to do something differently and rejoice that we are creating a brain that is going to support us long into the future to have the life that we really want to have.

> **ON THIS BRIGHT DAY,**
> I WILL NOTICE THE TRIGGER OF PAST CONDITIONING,
> BREATHE, AND MAKE AN EMPOWERED CHOICE.

October

TRUST THE PROGRAM

We don't know who discovered water,
but we're certain it wasn't a fish.
— JOHN CULKIN

After years of dieting, it can be difficult to trust another program for weight loss, let alone trust yourself to follow it. But you can trust the science, you can trust the thousands who have followed it successfully to a Bright Body and maintained that for years, and you can trust the part of you that found BLE, knew it was worth trying, and is still here.

Deeply trusting, whether ourselves or the program, is a process. We may not arrive at wholehearted trust quickly or easily. But a good proxy for deep trust is taking the necessary actions— just for this minute and this day—and allowing trust to grow. We come by our distrust honestly, and the protective parts of ourselves that learned to be on guard need us to be patient with them.

You can trust that you are in the right place at the right time and that your life is unfolding in a way that makes sense for your best and highest good. You can trust that working this program is something to be proud of.

ON THIS BRIGHT DAY,

I BECOME A BEGINNER AND TRUST THOSE WHO HAVE SUCCESSFULLY FOLLOWED THIS PLAN.

COMMITMENT OVER 51 PERCENT

> The purpose of discipline is to promote freedom.
> But freedom leads to infinity and infinity is terrifying.
> — HENRY MILLER

It is easier to do this program when we are fully committed to it, but the reality is that over the long term our commitment level is going to rise and fall like a sine wave. If we look back, there have probably been times when we were so head-over-heels committed to this program that our heart just sang from having found our solution. Then there were times when our recovery was hanging by a thread. But in those times, we can still tell that our commitment was over 51 percent because we are here right now. We are showing up.

Increasing our commitment by activating our tools is the investment we can make today to make sure that we are on the rise tomorrow.

ON THIS BRIGHT DAY,

I BUILD ON MY COMMITMENT THROUGH MY BRIGHT ACTIONS.

October 3
BEFRIEND THE BODY

Resilience is built into the cells of our bodies . . . [and] can be passed down from generation to generation.

— RESMAA MENAKEM

So many of us have been battling our bodies for years and may continue to berate ourselves for not losing weight fast enough. We have oriented toward our body as a project, and a fixer-upper at that. When we constantly try to change it, we are telling our body that it is not good enough. But that is not reality.

BLE presents an opportunity to work *with* our bodies, to love our bodies the way they are today, and to actively appreciate our health, our stamina, our resilience, and all the ways our bodies have been such loyal friends to us. Our bodies have withstood bingeing and restriction, overexercising, and complete statue-like sedentariness. Take this moment today to give deep thanks to the amazing vehicle of your soul, the one that has been with you every step of the way. Loving and befriending your body should not be postponed until you are at some ideal weight.

Choose to look at your body in a different way. Perhaps put lotion on every inch of your body in a loving way today. Find a part of your body that shows up for you every day and gets the job done without thanks or notice, and pour your awareness and gratitude into it. Do it right now. It is long overdue.

ON THIS BRIGHT DAY,

I WILL CELEBRATE THE GIFT OF MY BODY.

HEALTHIER WITH BLE

We must not, in trying to think about how we can make
a big difference, ignore the small daily differences we can
make which, over time, add up to big differences
that we often cannot foresee.

— MARIAN WRIGHT EDELMAN

As the years pass and we stay committed to this way of eating and living, the gifts we are giving ourselves gradually accumulate. Those who eat the BLE way report better sleep, which, combined with the removal of the inflammatory properties of sugar, allows the body to decrease inflammation and aching and helps alleviate certain conditions like insulin resistance and elevated cholesterol.

Living Bright is a gift to the people who want to see us live long, healthy lives and to everyone who benefits from every talent and capacity we have to give the world. By living this way, we will likely have hundreds, perhaps thousands, more healthy, vital days to offer. We often think of wanting to change the world by being of service; putting healthy food into our bodies consistently adds up to a major service that we can do for the world.

ON THIS BRIGHT DAY,

I WILL REVEL IN HOW EACH OF MY CELLS IS
BECOMING HEALTHIER.

THE 4 QUESTIONS

Never be afraid to sit awhile and think.
— LORRAINE HANSBERRY

We always need to be examining the foods we are eating and the ways we are eating them, continually taking inventory and asking ourselves questions. It is intrinsic to the dance of food recovery.

We are clear that we eliminate all sugar and flour, but when it comes to everything else, there is a lot of gray area around which food is recovery-based and which food might trigger us. It is different for different people and not always obvious.

If you want to run an experiment, then ask yourself these four questions for a few days in a row about the food, beverage, or way of eating that might be borderline: 1) Does it bring me peace? 2) Is it healthy? 3) Is it messing with my weight? 4) Is it escalating?

Plenty of people give up foods that are on the plan because they are too attached to them, their weight is escalating, or their mind is filled with food chatter between meals. Nuts and nut butters are a prime candidate. Melted cheese is another. We always need to be asking ourselves: *Is this working? Do I have peace?*

ON THIS BRIGHT DAY,

I WILL HONESTLY INVENTORY WHAT FOODS BRING ME PEACE.

October 6
MOTIVES MATTER

Try to be one of the people on whom nothing is lost.
— HENRY JAMES

In BLE, we do not eat foods processed with sugar and flour, but some foods that are minimally processed are allowed, such as nut butters and certain flour-free crackers. And some people in BLE bake using oats, eggs, bananas, and other BLE-friendly ingredients. Why we are eating each food makes the difference. Are we eating flourless crackers with hummus, say, simply because it is the quickest option and leads to no destabilization of our program? Or are we eating that because it is more pleasurable and our brain is looking to get a hit off it?

Notice if you are baking, making your food complicated, or including more processed foods regularly in your weekly menu, and see if you might be happier simplifying your food. If you find yourself having more food thoughts, feeling tempted, or even breaking your Lines, examine what you are eating and adjust. Honesty begins with the food. And when we become consistent about examining our motives around our food, it translates into examining our motives around our relationships and our actions.

ON THIS BRIGHT DAY,

I NOTICE MY MOTIVES WITH HONESTY AND INTEGRITY.

October 7
TRUE TREATS

Don't seek what you yearn for;
seek the source of the yearning.
— ADYASHANTI

Sweets are what most people mean when they suggest having a treat. Now that we are not eating sugar or flour, it is time to redefine what a treat is, listen deeply to what we truly want, and give ourselves the benefit of real pleasures.

Notice what you are craving—if it is sugar, you may want more sweetness in your life, and that can take the form of puppies and children or tenderness with those you love. If your old idea of a treat was something salty and crunchy, perhaps your true treat might be an adventurous outing to a new neighborhood and strolling around. Most of the time, the treat we really desire is rest, connection, or play. Take the time to discern just what you want and figure out what would serve as a satisfying treat.

ON THIS BRIGHT DAY,
I WILL SEEK ESPECIALLY TENDER MOMENTS,
BEAUTY, AND CONNECTION.

October 8
A BRIGHT BODY

Guided by my heritage of a love of beauty and a respect for strength—in search of my mother's garden, I found my own.
— ALICE WALKER

In the early days when the Bright Line Eating community was young and still forming, we focused a lot on goal weight and it did not serve us. People got hung up on the number. We saw people lose 100 or 150 pounds and have a hard time losing the last 5 pounds and feel like a failure. It was frustrating and ridiculous, really. The truth is that this journey has no endpoint and success is not defined by a number. First of all, not everybody wants to get down to a particular goal weight, or even thinks of their journey in those terms. And those of us who do need to be especially mindful to broaden our definition of success.

We talk about a Bright Body now because although it is true that weight loss is part of the equation for most people who are on a food recovery journey, your weight loss is unique to you. Sure, there are formulas that will give you guidelines, but it is really important that you think about what you would like to be able to do and *experience* in your body. If you want to take a long bike ride with your grandkids, that is a benchmark for your Bright Body. Maybe you would like to run a half marathon or do a pull-up, swim, or garden on your knees. Maybe you would like to dance without being self-conscious or shop in a store you haven't visited for years. However you decide to define it, BLE will get you there.

ON THIS BRIGHT DAY,

I WILL CELEBRATE WHATEVER A BRIGHT BODY MEANS TO ME.

October 9
ONLINE SUPPORT COMMUNITY

We cannot live only for ourselves. A thousand fibers connect us;
and among those fibers, as sympathetic threads, our actions run
as causes, and they come back to us as effects.

— HENRY MELVILL

Take the time to get to know others; post your stories, celebrations, and struggles; and comment and support others throughout the week. If you are worried about being sucked into the black hole of technology, put some boundaries around the amount of time or the time of day you log in. After all, now that you are eating BLE, you know how to put boundaries around things.

Whatever your take on technology, you will no doubt find that the love and support in the BLE community are exquisite and unparalleled, and there is so much wisdom and experience among the people who have been doing this before you. Also, your BLE identity is hard to form on your own. Immersing yourself in a community that already exists will help support your program.

These connections change lives, and we are blessed to live in a time when connecting with other human beings is so convenient and easy. The more deeply supported and connected we feel in this world, the happier we become, and the more energy we have.

ON THIS BRIGHT DAY,

I WILL CONNECT IN THE ONLINE SUPPORT COMMUNITY,
POST, AND OFFER SUPPORT.

October 10

NOTICE PATTERNS

You need only claim the events of your life to make yourself
yours. When you truly possess all you have been and done,
which may take some time, you are fierce with reality.

— FLORIDA SCOTT-MAXWELL

Behavior occurs in patterns, so noticing our patterns of connecting, disconnecting, following directions, rebelling, or resisting can be quite helpful in adjusting our habits to make BLE a lifelong identity and practice. The best way to notice patterns is to keep track of things, monitoring how we did *this* day. Otherwise, the brain remembers in aggregate, and the nuances of what actually occurred throughout the week will be lost in a glossy overview.

Create a checklist for yourself and ask, for example, on a scale from 1 to 10, how fierce (10) or nonexistent (1) are your food thoughts today? On a scale from 1 to 10, how deeply loved and connected are you feeling in the world today? Did you meditate? Did you write down your food the night before? Did you eat only and exactly that? Then once you have been able to look at the data, ask yourself: *Are there actions you could take based on that data?* The patterns will guide you on your Bright Journey.

ON THIS BRIGHT DAY,

I AM OPEN TO RECOGNIZING PATTERNS AND MAKING CHOICES.

October 11

PLAY

Just play. Have fun. Enjoy the game.
— MICHAEL JORDAN

Play is important. In her research, Brené Brown, Ph.D., has found that people who routinely play are more shame resilient—play being defined as any activity where we enjoy ourselves and lose track of time. If we routinely substituted eating NMF for the regenerative benefits of play, we have to relearn what a fun nonfood activity could be.

Perhaps we ate and watched TV because eating was the way we justified doing something relaxing. Learning that we do not need to eat in order to chill or take a break or have fun is important. Make a list of the things that would feel playful and give your inner Indulger something fun to do. If a part of you is resistant, get curious about why.

When it comes to deciding what to try, ask yourself the following questions: *What makes my heart sing? What brings real joy?* The invitation here is to reflect on what has really been fun for you in your life. Is it trying a pottery class? Taking up pickleball? Volunteering at an animal rescue? When do you get so lost in how much you are enjoying yourself that you lose track of time? Do more of that!

ON THIS BRIGHT DAY,

I TAKE MY NEED TO PLAY SERIOUSLY.

October 12

SETTLING OR COMPROMISE?

> If you have got a living force and you're not using it, nature kicks
> you back. The blood boils just like you put it in a pot.
>
> — LOUISE NEVELSON

Whenever we settle for something less than what our heart truly desires, we look for a consolation prize, and often in the past, that prize has been eating. We can shift the consolation prizes in our life to nonfood items *or* we can decide not to settle and really go for exactly what we want. The distinction is that settling involves some disappointment, whereas compromise involves some love.

We compromise on our vacation plans so that everyone is happy because we want everyone to be happy. We compromise on the new couch because everyone's perspective is important and we know that coming to a consensus reinforces our sense of teamwork and camaraderie. But if you are the only person making adjustments and you feel you are settling instead if compromising, allow your Bright Journey and the support you have found here to enable you to speak up and advocate for yourself. You do not have to settle.

ON THIS BRIGHT DAY,

I WILL NOTICE WITH CURIOSITY WHERE I MAY BE SETTLING.

NOT JUST A FOOD PLAN

[We] are not free when we are doing just what [we] like.
[We] are only free when [we are] doing what the
deepest self likes. And there is getting down to
the deepest self! It takes some diving.

— D. H. LAWRENCE

The reality is that Bright Line Eating goes way beyond a food plan. It is a set of habits. It is morning routines; it is evening routines. It is a community, and it is an identity that flows from belonging to that community. It is inner work. And all of that together makes long-term sobriety from sugar and flour possible.

Most people come to BLE to address their food and their weight, but when they work the full program, they find the benefits go far, far beyond those goals. They are transformed in every aspect of their lives. Their sense of identity changes to someone who takes care of themselves with love and respect, who is capable and strong. Their sense of connectedness is revolutionized as they build community. And their sense of what is possible bursts wide open. Yes, the food plan will change your body, but the program will change your life.

ON THIS BRIGHT DAY,

I WILL BE REALLY HONEST WITH MYSELF ABOUT
WHETHER I AM WORKING THE PROGRAM.

October 14

JOURNALING

When we write we begin to taste the texture of our own mind . . .
we come face-to-face with our own aloneness, sit in our own
loneliness. It is hard, painful, but it is real.

— NATALIE GOLDBERG

There are many ways of putting pen to paper in service of our Bright Transformation. There is writing down our food the night before, there is writing a gratitude list, and then there is journaling. Journaling, or writing our thoughts as they come to us for no other audience than ourselves, is a useful tool for listening to the inner emotions and ideas that have historically been stuffed down by food.

Research shows there is a cognitive difference between typing on a keyboard and writing longhand.[7] We unlock a different part of our mind, and what is often amazing is that when we put pen to paper, our words go in a direction entirely different than we had thought they might. By writing about our day, what has been working, what is in our heart, and what got under our skin, we externalize these moments and gain a new perspective on them.

On the BLE journey, your life and body are undergoing powerful changes and having a written record of this miracle is precious. Remember, you never have to show your journal to anyone else.

ON THIS BRIGHT DAY,

I WILL COMMIT MY THOUGHTS TO PAPER AND
SEE WHAT IS REVEALED.

October 15
EMOTIONAL STRETCH

When we close the door to our feelings, we close the door to the vital currents that energize and activate our thoughts and actions.
— GARY ZUKAV

Sometimes what feels like hunger is actually just emotional stretching. Now that we are not eating for comfort, when uncomfortable feelings arise, we have to develop new skills for coping with them. It can seem like a monumental task. But when we realize we only have to feel our one day's share, then it becomes much more manageable to be present with our feelings, acknowledge them, approach them with curiosity, and know that this too shall pass.

Most of us need practice, and it can feel scary, so we do not do it alone. We tell our friends and our loved ones what is going on. We post in the online community and absorb all the support we can, and together we ride the wave. We are building a new toolkit and rewiring the brain with new cue → response behavior patterns. Over time we become highly functional human beings with all sorts of coping skills that do not involve turning to food. You just need to not eat over your feelings—one minute at a time, one meal at a time, then one day at a time.

ON THIS BRIGHT DAY,

I WILL FEEL THE EMOTIONAL STRETCH AND
CELEBRATE THAT I AM NOT EATING OVER IT.

October 16

BLTS

We tell lies when we are afraid . . . afraid of what
we don't know, afraid of what others will think, afraid
of what will be found out about us. But every time we
tell a lie, the thing that we fear grows stronger.

— TAD WILLIAMS

Food addiction is actually twin addictions; there is the substance addiction, which we heal by giving up sugar and flour. And then there is the process addiction, the addiction to the act of eating itself. Bites, Licks, and Tastes (BLTs) may seem harmless, but they prevent the brain from healing the process addiction. Yes, even if it is Bright Line food. If it is more than our weighed portion or eaten between a meal, then it messes with our peace of mind and keeps alive and active the part of us that once grazed all day.

It is precision with the scale, meal timing, and no BLTs that helps us heal from the process addiction. We do not want a brain that is hounding us: *Did I get enough yet? Could I have a little bit more? How about another bite? How about a bite now? How about a little bit of that? Now?* We want freedom. So, train yourself early to not take BLTs. Graph it and chart it, monitor it on your Nightly Checklist, and learn to wait by delaying your gratification until you are sitting at the table. You will have so much more freedom than those few moments of impatient pleasure afford.

ON THIS BRIGHT DAY,

I WILL CLEAN UP MY LINES AND NOT FOOL MYSELF.

CONDIMENTS

I bought some powdered water,
but I don't know what to add.
— STEVEN WRIGHT

We use condiments freely in BLE, unless they are a significant source of nutrients, and then we weigh those as well
because those of us who are overeaters do not do well with the
idea of unlimited quantities of anything. Our use of condiments
offers an insight into how we are working our program, our emotional stability with our food, and our level of honesty with ourselves. If we are experiencing some Maintenance weight creep,
the way we are doctoring up our food could be the source of
those extra pounds. But there is nothing holy or righteous about
doing away with all seasoning to our food. Our food should be
delicious, and we should absolutely enjoy it.

Take a rigorous look at any seasonings or toppings you may
have become too attached to or might be overreliant on or excessively liberal with, and perhaps let them go for a week or two.
Simplify your food and detach from what might be lighting up
those old neural pathways.

ON THIS BRIGHT DAY,

I WILL BE JUDICIOUS WITH CONDIMENTS AND CURIOUS
ABOUT WHAT I SEEK FROM MY MEALS.

October 18
NUMBING

One must go through periods of numbness
that are harder to bear than grief.
— ANNE MORROW LINDBERGH

Anyone with neuropathy will tell you that there is nothing pleasant about numbing, but many of us used food, and bingeing in particular, to do just that. What we are learning to do in BLE is give ourselves periodic time off from our busy lives and legitimate concerns. Learning to take a true break without food to numb us can be challenging, and yet there is no shame in not "adulting" every single minute of every single day.

A long bubble bath, a book that does not actually "improve" our mind but entertains us nonetheless, a game on our phone, and some time watching a favorite show are all fine ways to give ourselves time off, within balance and reason. You will know when you have passed the point into numbing because you no longer enjoy what you are doing—just as we used to stop enjoying the food after the first few bites but continued until the bitter end of the container or the evening.

Today, see if you can allow yourself some essential restorative time to replenish your energy and enthusiasm while still maintaining presence.

ON THIS BRIGHT DAY,
I WILL SEEK RESPITE WITHOUT NUMBING.

October 19
DAILY REINFORCEMENT

Properly used, positive reinforcement
is extremely powerful.

— B. F. SKINNER

Reinforcing your identity as a Bright Lifer should be done daily, especially in the beginning when it is so new. Even when we become experienced, successful Bright Lifers, we recommit to our program in three main ways. First, we keep our daily habits fresh to reinforce that we do this because it works, because it is nourishing, and because it is who we are. Second, we handle our food. We write it down, and then eat only and exactly that. Third, we stay closely connected with others who are walking this path.

We can look for erosion in any of these three areas. Are we not doing our daily habits faithfully? Have our food behaviors gotten sloppy? Are we not fully connecting with other people on this journey? Conversely, if we are working this program faithfully, can we take a moment to see how much we are doing each day (without much effort anymore) and celebrate that automaticity? Either way, on this day we can recommit to taking these three actions that reinforce our Bright Identity and our commitment to our Bright Transformation.

ON THIS BRIGHT DAY,

I ATTEND TO THE SMALL ACTIONS THAT
REINFORCE MY BRIGHT IDENTITY.

ENLARGEMENT OVER COMFORT

Freedom lies in being bold.

— ROBERT FROST

When we first get Bright, everything can feel like a stretch. That is natural because we are abandoning a whole suite of automatic ways to handle the day, handle life, handle food, and handle food preparation, and consciously replacing them with a host of new behaviors that are completely unfamiliar to our brain. It is an earthquake. But as our new way of living takes root and builds new fiber tracts in the brain, these changes start to feel more familiar and comfortable, and that is a good thing.

However, as people with brains that are attuned to using sugar, flour, and excess quantities of food as a means of comfort, we need to continue to stretch ourselves in our recovery and perhaps engage where we would have avoided doing so in the past.

Try exploring one new thing every week. Talk to a stranger in BLE and make a new friend. Walk a different route on your daily walk. Listen to a different coach and discover your shared experiences. Keep broadening your Bright horizons.

ON THIS BRIGHT DAY,

I STEP OUT OF MY COMFORT ZONE
AND TRY SOMETHING NEW.

October 21

EASE

Try to be like the turtle—at ease in your own shell.
— BILL COPELAND

Some of us have been so caught up in struggling with our weight, debating food thoughts, and fighting our urges that a life of ease may seem unimaginable. Yet it is true that ease is available, though it may take some getting used to.

Start today by noticing where you are feeling ease in your body: Which muscles feel good? Where are you not tense? How deeply can you breathe? And then notice areas of ease in your mind: What are you not worrying about? Where is there a sense of well-being? What relationships are you enjoying?

We are so accustomed to finding where the problem is, we may well overlook huge swaths of ease that exist. Paying attention, noting them, and basking in them will allow ease to become more and more the norm.

ON THIS BRIGHT DAY,
I ACCEPT THE EASE IN MY LIFE AND
TAKE A MOMENT TO SAVOR IT.

October 22

KINDNESS

Wherever there is a human being,
there is an opportunity for a kindness.
— LUCIUS ANNAEUS SENECA

When it comes to how we treat ourselves, kindness is the virtue that tends to be in short supply. How often do we deny ourselves the kindness we offer to others? Sometimes an Inner Critic has become so blended with our self-talk that we hear judgment without anyone else expressing it. That is why it is important to take a look at that Inner Critic in the same spirit of kindness we often offer others. After all, it is trying to help us.

Our Inner Critic wants us to fit in, to win other people's love and affection and acceptance. It may have a misguided and unhelpful way of trying to get us there, but we must feel compassion for that Inner Critic because it absorbed someone else's judgment long ago and turned it inward. We can change all that now by extending ourselves the kindness of following our Bright Lines. Eventually, as we grow in our BLE identity, that level of self-care and kindness naturally becomes who we are and what we do.

ON THIS BRIGHT DAY,

I ACT FROM KINDNESS, ESPECIALLY TOWARD MYSELF.

October 23
AMAZE YOURSELF

If you ask me what I came to do in this world, I, an artist,
will answer you: I am here to live out loud!
— ÉMILE ZOLA

Taking on an issue we have struggled with throughout our life is a huge challenge and a great opportunity. To succeed, we are called upon to do things differently—because we want to get different results. Toward that end, we will be using new emotional and mental muscles that have perhaps been dormant. We will try new ways of being in the world.

The first step for all of us is to "come all the way in and sit all the way down." To surrender ourselves to this path. We do not have to believe that it will work. All we need to do is commit ourselves to it today.

You will be amazed when you walk through the world without using food as a coping device and learn to celebrate this new, or perhaps more original and authentic, you. You are embarking on a bold and audacious journey to blow yourself away and accept a level of Brightness, vitality, and opportunity in your life that you have never had before. It is a bold and wonderful thing to do.

ON THIS BRIGHT DAY,
I WELCOME ALL I DO NOT KNOW AND AM EASILY AMAZED.

October 24

PROGRESS

Move at the pace of guidance.
— CHRISTINA BALDWIN

On the recovery journey, progress is incremental. Our habits improve incrementally, our weight releases incrementally, and our sense of well-being is restored incrementally. It behooves us to become skilled at noting it. If we have only got our eye on outcomes, then every point along the path from A to Z becomes "not Z" because it is not the outcome. That mindset will pave the way for a slow and unhappy journey. We can avoid this by celebrating and taking note of all the small moments of change and progress along the way.

Look back for a moment. How far have you come? Take stock of all the ways you have already changed. Be sure to pay attention to the progress of things that are noted by their absence, like a lack of impatience, a lack of cigarettes, or other habits or inclinations that have fallen away. Perhaps put pen to paper to capture the changes and celebrate your progress.

ON THIS BRIGHT DAY,
I WILL TAKE STOCK OF HOW FAR I HAVE COME.

October 25

COMPLEXITY

I should like to insist that nearly all the
important questions, the things we ponder in our
profoundest moments, have no answers.
— JACQUETTA HAWKES

It may be tempting to analyze ourselves and seek the complicated reasons we have had a particular relationship with food that has made us unhappy or overweight. Sometimes that self-knowledge is useful and interesting, but truly, we overeat for two reasons: 1) because we are food addicts who are high on the Susceptibility Scale or 2) because our brains are hijacked once highly addictive food is in our bodies, and we eat more than we intended, no matter where we land on the Susceptibility Scale.

Food addiction can turn our brains into tangled balls of yarn. The way to straighten out that tangled ball of yarn is one meal at a time. While we cannot think our way into right action, we can act our way into right thinking. It is through action, not overthinking, that progress happens.

ON THIS BRIGHT DAY,

I EMBRACE THE MYSTERY OF LIFE AND TURN MY
ATTENTION TO THE NEXT RIGHT ACTION.

THE UNIVERSE HAS YOUR BACK

The winds of grace blow all the time.
All we need to do is set our sails.
— RAMAKRISHNA

Instinctively, we can find evidence for whatever hypothesis we are testing at the moment. If we think the world is out to get us, we are sure to find ways in which that is true. If we feel like the world is on our side, sure enough, there is plenty of evidence for that as well.

Something brought you here, to this community, to this opportunity for a life free from the suffering of food and weight struggles. Many of us have come to believe that some force is conspiring in our favor. Leaning in to that idea when the road gets challenging can make all the difference. Entertain the idea that a higher power, the universe, or others in this community have your back. Allowing yourself to tune into whatever you feel wants the best for you will bring you a bit more ease and comfort on this journey.

ON THIS BRIGHT DAY,

I FEEL DEEPLY SUPPORTED BY THE LOVING UNIVERSE.

October 27
ALL IS FUNDAMENTALLY WELL

Inside yourself or outside, you never have to change
what you see, only the way you see it.
— THADDEUS GOLAS

A beautiful mantra to have at the ready whenever you feel your peace of mind ebbing away is "All is fundamentally well."

It is a great reminder that in the big scheme of things, everything is working out for you. No matter the challenges you are facing today . . . you are alive! You are doing BLE! You are loved! You have talents and gifts, unique contributions to make, and the time and space to focus on your health. To tune into any of these wonderful blessings, all you have to do is notice them, and they are there. Keep "all is fundamentally well" in mind and watch everything fall into place.

ON THIS BRIGHT DAY,

I WILL TRY ON THE PERSPECTIVE THAT ALL IS
FUNDAMENTALLY WELL, NO MATTER WHAT.

LEAVE NOTHING TO CHANCE

Quality is doing it right when no one is looking.
— HENRY FORD

Even the most experienced airline pilot uses a checklist before every single flight. Every time. That is because it is not enough to assume experience will ensure safety. Such is also the case with recovery. Even if we have eaten the same thing for breakfast for a year, writing it down the night before and committing it to ourselves or another human being leaves nothing to chance.

Using your checklists to ensure you have done what it takes to protect your Lines makes you the most responsible pilot of your Bright Journey. Then with your instrument panel in perfect working shape, you truly can fly.

ON THIS BRIGHT DAY,
I THOROUGHLY WORK MY BLE PROGRAM TO
ENSURE A SMOOTH JOURNEY.

October 29
CENTERING

Go into your own ground and learn to know yourself there.
— MEISTER ECKHART

There is a saying, "No one ever falls off the middle of the wagon." Whatever metaphor we prefer, our inner work is to remain in the center of the BLE lane, in the middle of the community, and hopeful about our progress. It is easier to keep moving forward from the center than the margins, where old feelings of unworthiness and not belonging and self-pity may lurk. The goal of the BLE life is to remain centered under all conditions because now we have tools other than food to keep us grounded.

In the early days of the Bright Line Eating movement, we took the time at the start of every coaching call to do a brief centering exercise, often focusing on our breath, with our feet on the floor. There is a parallel between centering ourselves with our breath, which is something we learn through meditation, and staying centered in the BLE community itself. These are the twin pillars of our rootedness. They keep us centered not just in our Bright Line Eating program, but happy, thriving, peaceful, and calmly centered in our lives as a whole.

ON THIS BRIGHT DAY,
I MOVE TOWARD CENTER.

October 30
BOUNDARIES

Whereas I formerly believed it to be my bounden
duty to call other persons to order, I now admit
that I need calling to order myself.

— CARL JUNG

Boundaries differ from barriers. Barriers are walls that close us off from others, while boundaries are a clear delineation of what we need and how we live our lives. It is important to learn how to hold our boundaries without walling ourselves off from the people who love us. Our community becomes one of the greatest gifts of this program, and being authentic, vulnerable, and open with others can be the path to deep and nourishing friendships.

Boundaries can also help us to maintain close relationships with people outside the program who may need to be educated about how to support our recovery. For example, we will not eat the NMF served at a family meal, but we do want to connect with our family. While it is paramount for us to have boundaries in our recovery, in BLE, we want to avoid barriers to close connections.

ON THIS BRIGHT DAY,

I KEEP MY BOUNDARIES FIRM WHILE I RELEASE
MY BARRIERS AND MOVE INTO CONNECTION.

October 31
TRICK OR TREAT

If human beings had genuine courage,
they'd wear their costumes every day of the year,
not just on Halloween.
— DOUGLAS COUPLAND

Halloween in many countries is a time for NMF, not just for children who come costumed to the front door shouting "trick or treat," but also for adults at parties, in the office, or as they are handing out NMF to little ghosts and goblins. Remember that eating NMF tonight is a huge trick, no treat.

It is a lie that we can have a holiday off from the BLE food plan. This is the way we live, and our brains and bodies will react addictively to sugar or flour no matter what date the calendar says. As always with any food-based occasion, if we do not want to partake, there is absolutely nothing wrong with that. Some of us give out coins instead. Or leave a bowl of NMF on our porch for kids to help themselves to. Or if we want to skip it altogether, we keep the lights off and watch a movie. But above all, we are aware of old patterns and habits today and take care that we feel fully supported by our community if we are going to handle NMF tonight.

ON THIS BRIGHT DAY,

I WILL REMEMBER THAT "ONE IS TOO MANY
AND A THOUSAND NEVER ENOUGH" AND LEAN INTO
THE BLE COMMUNITY FOR STRENGTH.

November

November 1

THE NEXT RIGHT THING

You cannot make yourself feel something you
do not feel, but you can make yourself do right
in spite of your feelings.

— PEARL S. BUCK

When we feel overwhelmed by all the tools required for our recovery, it is helpful to simply do what is next and not look too far into the future. Most likely the *next* action is fairly easy to discern. But what about the *right* action?

When we do face uncertainty about the next right thing, it is important to release our needs and expectations and just breathe and trust that all will unfold as it should.

In stillness we look for how our intuition is leading us from the place of our Authentic Self. Staying in touch with that place from within provides the confidence and courage we need to take action. Try to get calm, clear, connected, confident, courageous, and (most of all) curious. And then from that place ask, *What seems like the next right thing?* It usually turns out to be something simple—starting to prepare our next Bright meal, taking out the trash, or calling a friend who needs support.

ON THIS BRIGHT DAY,

I WILL TUNE INTO THE ENERGY OF MY AUTHENTIC SELF
AND DO THE NEXT RIGHT THING.

CREATE GOOD HABITS

Good habits are worth being fanatical about.
— JOHN IRVING

Building good habits from the start is so much easier than dismantling and replacing bad habits later. A stack of good habits eventually becomes the structure within which keeping our Lines Bright takes place, and those habits will raise us above the danger and destruction zone so we never have to eat to cope. When we faithfully stick to our habits, and do them at the same time each day, cued by the same precursor, we build automaticity. Automaticity frees up our cognitive resources so that it feels like we are living an incredibly effective and productive life filled with self-care, healthy eating, and tons of discipline—but it is all happening with little to no cognitive effort. The repetition that we establish today will breed the ease of tomorrow.

ON THIS BRIGHT DAY,

I COMMIT TO MY HABITS AND LAY A STRONG FOUNDATION.

FLEXIBILITY

I can't understand why people are frightened of new ideas. I'm
frightened of the old ones.

— JOHN CAGE

You may be surprised after some time passes without sugar
and flour how much more physically flexible you are because
inflammation has left your joints. But what is it to be emotionally and intellectually flexible?

Letting go of immediate reactions, judgments, and critiques
creates space for wonder and inquiry, and that gives us room to
take in information and see what fits and what does not. Having a flexible framework for many of our habits and the way we
show up in our community means offering ourselves compassion
when we don't do things perfectly.

In recovery we coexist in a community with people who hold
very different ideas than us, both in their outside lives, such as
politically, and within Bright Line Eating, such as whether they
are plant-based or omnivores and also how they work their program. But we join as One on our Bright Line Eating journey, supporting one another with love and compassion. We can offer that
flexibility to others in the world knowing there are truly good,
soulful, heartfelt people who believe differently than we do about
matters we hold dear. We can return again and again to the truth
that our similarities are more significant than our differences.

ON THIS BRIGHT DAY,

I WILL HAVE THE FLEXIBILITY TO TRY ON A NEW
IDEA OR PERSPECTIVE.

COMFORT IN OUR BODY

In anything at all, perfection is finally attained not
when there is no longer anything to add, but when there
is no longer anything to take away, when a body
has been stripped down to its nakedness.

— ANTOINE DE SAINT-EXUPÉRY

Wanting to feel comfortable in our body is a reason many come to recovery in the first place. Many of us who are starting from bigger numbers experience marked milestones of comfort, like being able to cross our legs or fit in an airplane seat without a seatbelt extender or slide easily into a booth in a restaurant. But even those who had little to no weight to lose will likely notice increased comfort in their body as their brains, guts, and nervous systems heal and as inflammation recedes and sleep improves.

Pay attention to the small shifts that occur as you grow more comfortable in your body, in your clothing, and in your movement. Notice your expanding ease, and do not wait until you are in your Bright Body weight range to celebrate those blessings.

ON THIS BRIGHT DAY,

I EXPRESS GRATITUDE FOR THE STAMINA, STRENGTH,
AND HEALTH OF MY BODY.

November 5
FEEL IT ALL

Life is full of beauty. Notice it. Notice the bumble bee, the small child, and the smiling faces. Smell the rain, and feel the wind.
— ASHLEY SMITH

As we slow down and experience life without sugar, flour, and quantities as a crutch, we are likely to notice feelings coming up, feelings we used to eat over. The challenge and the gift we have before us now is just to feel them. If we feel sad, we let ourselves cry. If we feel fear, we name it—and feel it. If we feel embarrassment, we own it—and feel it. We even need to learn to allow joy, because we may have habitually turned to food to celebrate, when truly food was muting our joy.

Developing a practice of feeling our feelings and utilizing new coping strategies is going to be a big job for us right now. When we need support with these feelings, we can come to the community. We can use writing as a tool. We can call a friend. We can book a therapy session. And we can pray or meditate. But feeling the appropriate feeling at the appropriate time is one of the biggest gifts of this Bright Journey.

When we stuff down our feelings, they can come out sideways months or even years later in therapy sessions or in inexplicable bursts of anger. But when we feel our feelings in the moment, they pass like a weather system, and we emerge fresh and healthy.

ON THIS BRIGHT DAY,
I ALLOW MYSELF TO FEEL WHATEVER I FEEL,
KNOWING I CAN HANDLE IT.

November 6
PLAN FOR SUCCESS

This is one of the glories of humans, the inventiveness
of the human mind and the human spirit: Whenever life
doesn't seem to give us vision, we create one.

— LORRAINE HANSBERRY

If you have a history of failed diets, you may understandably approach BLE with a great deal of skepticism. The good news is that you do not have to believe this will work for it to work. You just have to do it. However, we invite you to plan for success and envision yourself having one Bright Day after another, doing whatever it takes to lay your head on the pillow after a successful day. Seeing yourself losing weight, navigating obstacles with grace, and immersing yourself in this loving community will help you learn how to do so.

Conversely, take a moment to imagine the moments when it will be hard, when you will have a craving, and when you will need to do something different than pick up the food. You will need to use a tool or get online in the support community and post that you are struggling. Imagine what is most likely to take you down, and then imagine yourself meeting that challenge head-on in a different way than you used to in the past. That is the type of visualization that is going to make a difference: envisioning the setbacks along the way and how you are going to overcome them. So go ahead, let yourself succeed at this.

ON THIS BRIGHT DAY,

I IMAGINE THE SUCCESS I WILL HAVE AND LEAN INTO IT.

HOLIDAYS

Character is doing the right thing when nobody's looking.
— J. C. WATTS

At heart, holidays are gatherings of beloved people. Learning to focus on the social aspects of any holiday, or the religious aspects if that is our orientation, or the communal connections if it is a shared or national holiday, becomes a skill that serves us well and may perhaps even become a model for others.

Holidays can ultimately become automatic, and even easy, if we train our brain right from the beginning to not expect any deviation. We make up for what initially will feel like a loss of the part of us that really loved to indulge on holidays with the nourishment we can get out of real, meaningful human connection and being of service to others.

It is important to lay a strong foundation with your first holiday season because you will reap the rewards every holiday season thereafter. When we stay Bright and honor ourselves with our Bright food and give our heart and soul to the occasion, we will have so much to celebrate and be truly thankful for when our head hits the pillow at night.

ON THIS BRIGHT DAY,

I CELEBRATE BY FOLLOWING MY PLAN REGARDLESS OF WHAT OTHERS ARE EATING.

BLE-FRIENDLY KITCHEN

*The aspects of things that are most important to us are
hidden because of their simplicity and familiarity.*
— LUDWIG WITTGENSTEIN

Before beginning BLE, we invite everyone who lives alone to inventory their kitchen and rid their fridge and pantry of non-BLE foods. Everyone should give themself the benefit of a safe environment from which to navigate an outer world that is not under their control. But many of our Bright Lifers have families who eat NMF, especially children who need a lot of starch in their diet.

It is still possible to set your kitchen up Bright. Perhaps have a separate cupboard for their snacks or an area of the fridge where they keep their NMF. Or an area of the fridge where *you* keep *your* Bright food. Even something as simple as that will help your eyes go just to where your food will be. It is important that we advocate for ourselves and that we set up our kitchen clean and strong. No matter where you are on your journey, it is a good idea to revisit this aspect of your program regularly.

ON THIS BRIGHT DAY,

I CELEBRATE THE CLEAN LINES IN MY KITCHEN
AND THE BRIGHT LINES IN MY MENU.

ANCHOR HABITS

I have resolved to grow old, naturally and gracefully,
content in the knowledge that the greatest intellects
are the homeliest ones, and that the height of
sophistication is simplicity.
— CLARE BOOTH LUCE

Whenever we feel overwhelmed by how many tools, practices, and habits there are to put in place for a successful
BLE journey, it helps to just pick one morning and one evening
habit that will anchor our identity as a Bright Lifer. Eventually,
when that feels automatic and we feel very nourished and replenished by doing it, we can add another. The completion of
one anchor habit becomes the cue to start the next action, and
suddenly we have a habit stack.

Many people find meditation is a good anchor habit for the
morning; and reading, journaling, or making a gratitude list can
be a good anchor habit for the evening. Every person is free to
pick the habit that most nourishes them, that makes the most
sense to them, or feels the most doable for whatever reason. So if
you are struggling to put those Bright routines in place, start with
one thing you can commit to consistently and go from there.

ON THIS BRIGHT DAY,
I FOCUS ON THE MOST IMPORTANT ACTIONS
THAT KEEP MY LINES BRIGHT.

November 10
SHIELDS UP

Through vigilance, restraint, and control the wise will construct an island that no flood will overcome.
— GAUTAMA BUDDHA

We all run the gauntlet of food cues every day, even just driving to work. Once we get to work, there might be NMF in the break room, NMF on offer at lunch, and a slew of food cues to drive past on the way home. The reason we use BLE tools every single day, even when it does not feel like we need them, is that we want to keep our shields up for those times when we could be ambushed by NMF, particularly when our willpower is already depleted.

When in recovery from any addiction, there is the daily maintenance that we all do, the little habits that keep the shields in good repair and create a force field that repels thoughts of the first bite, smoke, snort, or drink. But when we stop doing our habits and fall out of connection with our community and friends in recovery, our shield slowly goes down.

It may not seem like doing your morning meditation or filling out your Nightly Checklist is the equivalent of polishing your armor, but that is exactly what it is. Keep your defenses strong and you will be victorious.

ON THIS BRIGHT DAY,

I KEEP MY SHIELD UP EVEN IF THERE ARE NO PARTICULAR THREATS ON THE HORIZON.

November 11

DO NOT FEED EMOTIONS

Feelings are often interpreted as cravings.
— ELENE LOECHER

Emotions are part of being human, but growing up many of us had little help in feeling them, naming them, and reacting to them. Nor did we have models of adults feeling the full range of human emotions, expressing them appropriately, and allowing them to pass through. Those of us who ate emotionally learned to stuff these emotions with a bite of something, preferably something that offered a quick hit of dopamine and allowed us to chill out, numb out, or bliss out.

When crisis comes, as it does in all lives, many people turn to NMF and NMD to self-soothe over the anxiety, stress, and fear. It takes a lot of bravery to allow uncomfortable emotions and permit them to have their essential space and time. It is absolutely okay to not be okay every minute of every day. As the saying goes: I am not okay, you are not okay, and that's okay. Just for today, we are learning how to give our emotions respect, not food.

ON THIS BRIGHT DAY,
I TUNE INTO MY FEELINGS AND TURN TO SUPPORT
RATHER THAN FOOD.

SAY YES TO THE INVITATION

---

*I don't want to get to the end of my life and find
that I lived just the length of it.
I want to have lived the width of it as well.*

— DIANE ACKERMAN

Life is always inviting us toward being our healthiest, best selves. Sometimes we heed the invitation and sometimes we do not even hear it. Other times we ignore it or actively say no. Sometimes we do not feel ready. Other times we are afraid of success or transformation. Or maybe we do not feel worthy. Perhaps we are afraid of what other people might think if we shine that Bright.

But playing small does not serve the world. The fact that you are here means you are ready to commit with your whole self. So while there may be plenty more work to do, if you have received the invitation, you are ready enough to say yes and start on this journey.

ON THIS BRIGHT DAY,

I WILL SAY YES TO LIVING FULLY TO THE EDGES
OF MY BRIGHTEST LIFE.

ASK FOR WHAT YOU WANT

Leap and the net will appear.

— JULIA MARGARET CAMERON

A lot of us learned to play small in all kinds of ways growing up, to not be a bother, to not take up space, to not need anything. As we let go of distracting ourselves with food, we might find parts of ourselves making their wants and needs and preferences known, and we can learn to advocate for them.

As we express our needs in restaurants, at home, and at other gatherings, we will develop the muscles to ask for what we want in nonfood areas as well. We will learn to be explicit in our requests and give others the opportunity to meet our needs by communicating them clearly.

Not only are we landing in a Bright Body; we are using words to create the future we may have wanted for a lifetime.

ON THIS BRIGHT DAY,

I ALLOW MYSELF TO ASK FOR WHAT I WANT,
AND LET GO OF THE OUTCOME.

November 14

BOREDOM

*Boredom, anger, sadness, or fear are not "yours,"
not personal. They are conditions of the human mind.
They come and go. Nothing that comes and goes is you.*
— ECKHART TOLLE

People new to BLE often worry about becoming bored with the food. *Isn't it hard to never have NMF and what about all the new products the food industry is always introducing? Won't I miss out and get bored eating whole food all the time?* But we really are wired to keep our food simple. Research shows that our ancestors and people in present-day hunter-gatherer tribes eat very few foods. Often, they get more than 50 percent of their calories from just one food. It is only in our modern world of excessive sensory stimulation that this simplicity can translate to boredom. But as James Clear suggests, to master anything, you have to fall in love with boredom. Do not derail your program to make your food more interesting.

When we look at what is available in life, exciting food is a poor proxy for genuine thrill. Life can be so much bigger and more exciting than what we put in our stomach. When we release trying to generate all our joy through taste, we awaken to the true promise of a life of new and exciting experiences.

ON THIS BRIGHT DAY,
I EXPLORE NEW WAYS TO FEEL EXCITEMENT.

HOURGLASS

Life shrinks or expands in proportion to one's courage.
— ANAÏS NIN

It is natural for a Bright Transformation to have an hourglass shape, meaning that we start off from a history of a broad, freewheeling, *I can eat anything I want, anytime* mentality. But that did not work for us in all kinds of ways, so now we have arrived here. And as we first get sober from addictive eating, it can seem like our world narrows, which can feel like a form of deprivation. For some of us, that narrowing can be so extreme that it feels like we are confined to a very small box. But if we stay Bright and we stay the course, automaticity starts to build, our brains are rewired, and our experiences open back up until we gradually reintroduce travel, social experiences, restaurants, and all the things that we had left behind. Our life becomes expansive again, and this time without all the negative consequences of excessive eating.

If you are in a period of constriction, know that you are actually in a sort of birth canal, soon to be born to the freest life possible. And if you know someone who is in that place now, share with them that life is going to open up again soon and be greater than they ever could have imagined. Because once we have invested the time in that cramped space, we will have the strength to remain Bright no matter the circumstance.

ON THIS BRIGHT DAY,
I ACKNOWLEDGE THAT MY WORLD MUST SHRINK
BEFORE IT CAN EXPAND.

ALIGN WITH INSPIRATION

There are two ways of spreading light;
to be the candle or the mirror that reflects it.
— EDITH WHARTON

Inspiration is a filling of the spirit, a fullness in the heart, a lightness of being, and a palpable sense of hope. On this recovery journey, we get to choose whom to spend time with, whom we want in our life on a daily basis, and whom we invite to be a Buddy or a Mastermind Group member. When you are deciding who should be in your circle of support, pay attention to who inspires you. It may not only be the people who are keeping their Lines super Bright. It may be the person who is so clearly *unstoppable* that you know it is just a matter of time before their Lines shine too.

Surround yourself with people who inspire you; apprentice yourself to them as you learn how they work this program. Know that the part of you that is drawn to them is your Authentic Self, and you are already living there, right alongside them.

ON THIS BRIGHT DAY,
I DRAW CLOSE TO THOSE WHO INSPIRE ME.

November 17

SPACING MEALS

The only way of discovering the limits
of the possible is to venture a little way past
them into the impossible.
— ARTHUR C. CLARKE

In BLE, we eat our meals four to six hours apart, leaving a nice long window of fasting between supper and breakfast the next day to give our bodies enough time to empty out and for autophagy, the miraculous process of cellular repair, to kick in. This can feel quite scary and excruciating to those of us who used to eat every hour or so, never allowing the body to grow hungry, eating ahead of time in case we might get hungry later. But fasting is beneficial both from a physical perspective and a spiritual one.

Fasting is one of the common denominators among all the world's major religions. There is something holy and reverent and precious about the emptiness between meals; it is in that spaciousness that inspiration strikes as we realign ourselves and the small voice of wisdom can come visit.

ON THIS BRIGHT DAY,

I ATTUNE TO THE SPACE BETWEEN MEALS AND
STAY OPEN TO WHAT I MIGHT DISCOVER THERE.

PROTECT YOUR LINES

It doesn't take willpower to avoid the thing
that is sure to ruin my life; it just takes a fierce,
overriding desire to not ruin my life.

— KRISTI COULTER

We quickly learn that unless our Lines are Bright, nothing else in our lives really goes as well as it could. And our history shows that most often, eating outside the Bright Lines makes us downright miserable. In other words, making our recovery the priority and doing whatever it takes to get to bed squeaky clean Bright makes everything else in life better.

Perhaps you have started BLE and stayed consecutively Bright from the beginning. If so, biggest hug and huge high five! That is truly awesome and such a gift. On the other hand, perhaps you had a good beginning but have wavered and Rezoomed in fits, stringing a few days together before going off the Lines again. The next time you have a Bright Day (and you can restart your day at any time, so why not the next meal?), savor that Brightness and do what it takes the next day to have it again.

It so helps to be clear: Bright Lines are the foundation for everything your heart desires and for you to soar as the person you want to be in this world. Treat them as such.

ON THIS BRIGHT DAY,

I WILL SUMMON THE INNER STRENGTH AND OUTER SUPPORT TO FOLLOW THE PLAN NO MATTER WHAT.

November 19

A LIFE LIVED ELSEWHERE

Addiction is a life lived elsewhere.
— BILL ALEXANDER

When we are into the food, eating outside of meals, consuming the sugar and flour that are addictive substances in our bodies and brains, we are by definition not in the present moment, nor are we living the truth of ourselves.

It is okay to want a break from life from time to time. That is what sleep gives us, and TV, our smartphones, focusing on someone else, and getting into the zone of a creative act. But if we are checking out multiple times a day, we are missing the gift of being alive, because the only point of connection is in the present. Our job in recovery is to relearn how to be present to all that life offers up—the beauty and the struggle—without checking out. But we do not relearn this alone.

We build up this new skill in community with fellow learners and wise experts, those who walk alongside us and those who have walked ahead and laid the path. Pay attention today—what do you hear? What do you notice? We have four other senses begging for our attention. Let them feast on life.

ON THIS BRIGHT DAY,

I WILL STAY PRESENT AND NOTICE WHAT IT FEELS
LIKE TO BE RIGHT HERE IN THIS MOMENT.

November 20
GROWING UP

To mature is in part to realize that while
complete intimacy and omniscience and power
cannot be had, self-transcendence, growth,
and closeness to others are nevertheless
within one's reach.

— SISSELA BOK

It is hard to acknowledge, but most of us need to grow up more than we have. Growing up means taking responsibility for ourselves, and not blaming others for our former eating patterns, any current breaks in our program, or any unhappiness we are experiencing. Our eating often comes from a place of adolescent rebellion or childish impulsivity that, once we are Bright, we have to address.

Even if the rebellious teenager was legitimately pushing back against an overly authoritarian figure or system or if that impulsive child really did need to grab what they wanted because their needs might not have been provided for, part of growing up means reparenting, as it were, the wounded, rebellious, and young parts of ourselves that need our attention. They do not need anyone else anymore. They need us. Get curious, inquire, and listen for an answer. The adult, healed, whole part of you has been waiting to share for a long time!

ON THIS BRIGHT DAY,

I NOTICE WHERE I NEED TO MATURE AND
WELCOME THE CHALLENGE.

November 21
PRUNING

I'm a big fan of editing and keeping only
the interesting bits in.
— SARAH VOWELL

Pruning, in horticultural terms, means cutting something to facilitate growth. Dead leaves, too many branches, and sprouts too close together are all pruned to allow a plant to grow to its fullest capacity.

When we first start on this food recovery journey, it can feel like we are giving up too much. But it is important to remember that the plant that receives the most thorough pruning develops the most beautiful blossoms come spring and summer.

Although it feels like an extreme form of pruning, letting go of the foods and the eating behaviors that do not serve us anymore really benefits us in the end. So, too, with food thoughts. Prune them immediately. Do not let them take root in your mind so they become an obsession. Snip them away immediately and your mind will blossom.

ON THIS BRIGHT DAY,
I FOCUS ON WHAT I *DO* WANT AND LET
EVERYTHING ELSE FALL AWAY.

DREAM

Don't settle for little dreams.
— JUDY BALLARD

For many of us, losing weight was our primary dream for most of our lives. Every time we thought of trying to become a better version of ourselves, the first item on the to-do list was getting the excess weight off. And then we would dream and fantasize about that goal weight and how it would feel. But the truth is that the dream of being thin is a poor proxy for the reality of leading a rich and fulfilling life of wonderful relationships, meaningful service, higher purpose, and creative pursuits. A lot of us just settled for far too long, for far too little, and used food to anesthetize ourselves to the reality of what we were giving up.

Learning to rediscover those dreams, our best vision of our future selves, will take some time. Give yourself the gift of inviting your stifled dreams forward, of listening, and of honoring them by laying a Bright path forward. And let us celebrate today that our Bright Transformation is about so much more than the weight—it is about the dreams of our whole heart and soul.

ON THIS BRIGHT DAY,

I EMBRACE MY HEART'S MOST CHERISHED
DREAMS FOR MY FUTURE.

November 23
BE TENDER WITH YOURSELF

There is no charm equal to tenderness of heart.
— JANE AUSTEN

There will be days during our BLE journey when we will be tempted to scold ourselves for not doing what we hoped we would. The harder life gets and the more the day asks us to show up, the more our inner Manager part wants to shift into overdrive and tackle the day with ferocity. But sometimes we need to sense when being gentle, taking it slow, and having a heart of tender compassion for ourselves would actually be better.

Counterintuitively, we can often get more done when we slow down. And when we catch ourselves having an attitude that is less than positive, that is precisely the moment to offer ourselves compassion, to view ourselves with tenderness and curiosity. Nothing new grows in an environment of criticism; we do not change because we were judged. The more tender you are with yourself, the sooner old habits slip away and new ones become rooted.

ON THIS BRIGHT DAY,
I OFFER MYSELF TENDERNESS.

RETREAT

---

*In solitude the mind gains strength
and learns to lean upon itself.*
— LAURENCE STERNE

There are times when retreating feels natural, such as during winter or a period of depression or loss—the darkest times of the year when deep inner work can be nourished in solitude with a step back from ordinary life. Taking time each year to retreat, alone or with close friends or loved ones, serves our growth.

Typically, on retreat, one reflects on lessons, learnings, growth, and changes made or yearning to be made. Even daily, there may be a period when a retreat into our own inner landscape is nourishing. Meditation is one such retreat. If it is performed faithfully, it creates a little place deep inside where we can retreat at any moment—a place of sacred sanctuary inside us. Even if we have not yet started a daily meditation practice, we can breathe for a few moments and find that place.

Having a touchstone place to retreat to, a practice that allows you to unplug daily, or perhaps a teacher or community on retreat, can strengthen your program and your spirit.

ON THIS BRIGHT DAY,

I WILL TURN WITHIN AND REPLENISH.

SIMPLICITY

Everything should be as simple as it is,
but not simpler.
— ALBERT EINSTEIN

As the Shaker hymn says, "'Tis a gift to be simple. 'Tis a gift to be free." This song has endured and resonated for nearly 200 years because simplicity and freedom go hand in hand. While some people love trying new BLE-friendly recipes each week, the reality is that keeping our food simple allows the brain to relax and cue our body to release excess weight without resistance. For this reason, we want to fall in love with simplicity.

If our weight loss has stalled or if we are still plagued by breaks, cravings, and food thoughts, we are perhaps being called to eat simpler foods. And that can be a gift. Never confuse simple with boring. There is an art and genius to simplicity because it is often the hardest thing to achieve. Simplicity is a Brancusi sculpture, a line of Rumi poetry, or a Shaker box. There is reverence in simplicity, and it is this spirit we infuse into our program. When we keep our food simple, we make space for ease and grace.

ON THIS BRIGHT DAY,

I WELCOME A SIMPLE PATH.

November 26

LOVE

Love doesn't just sit there,
like a stone, it has to be made, like bread;
re-made all the time, made new.
— URSULA K. LE GUIN

Love is the most powerful force in the world. On the surface, it may seem like it has nothing to do with food addiction, but consuming only and exactly what we commit and following all four Bright Lines is a tremendous act of self-love. In giving ourselves this gift, we align our actions with our hopes and intentions, and thus become a vehicle for universal love. Eating this way is also a loving act to our planet as we remove ourselves from the industrial food complex that causes so much harm.

As you begin to shine with love for yourself and others, reflecting the love of this amazing BLE community, you will invite everyone you encounter to step into that sphere and bask in it for a time. This is what we were seeking when we ate excess food. This is what we thought NMF could provide. Yet it was a poor substitute for this love—this true, powerful, and pure energy.

ON THIS BRIGHT DAY,

I WILL SHARE MY LOVE WITH SOMEONE I MEET,
SOMEONE I REACH OUT TO,
AND SOMEONE I HAVE BEEN MISSING.

EAT ONLY AND EXACTLY THAT

My mother is a woman who speaks with her life
as much as with her tongue.
— KESAYA E. NODA

When we start swapping our food in the moment, we activate the part of our brain that makes impulse choices, and that part has been shown in studies to nearly always select higher-calorie foods.[8] Before we know it, we will be making heavier choices the norm and we will have a brain that is always looking for food to provide the next hit. That will stall our weight loss and is likely to lead to Maintenance weight creep later on.

And it starts small. While it might not seem like a big deal to swap asparagus for broccoli, even though you wrote the latter down on your food plan the night before, it does matter scientifically. When you eat what you committed, you strengthen your integrity. You become someone whose word matters. And you quiet the part of the brain that is looking for a solution in food. Often, the part of us that wants to swap foods is the one who called the shots when we were eating addictively. It is seductive. It will begin by saying, *Asparagus isn't NMF, so what's the harm?* Acting on that whim sets a precedent for the next whim that crosses our mind. It's better to have an automatic habit of eating only and exactly what we have already committed—it's a shield and firewall against such a rationale.

ON THIS BRIGHT DAY,

I KEEP MY WORD BY EATING ONLY AND
EXACTLY WHAT I HAVE COMMITTED.

WORKING IN GOOD TIMES

You have to be willing to go to war with yourself
and create a whole new identity.
— DAVID GOGGINS

There is no denying that doing BLE is work, especially at first. But we do not work our program just when we are in trouble; we do it every day because it is who we are. When we have had a stretch of very Bright Lines, it might be tempting to let up on all the daily work required, but that is precisely when it is important to double down and do everything with a whole heart.

Working in good times, doing the meditation, journaling, calling, listening, and offering support puts our roots much deeper into our BLE identity. When the day is smooth and our automaticity is working for us, following the plan is the insurance we build up for the days when we legitimately need to skip our meditation or condense our evening habit stack. The longer we do any action, the deeper that habit groove gets etched in our brain, and that is how identity shifts.

We want to take advantage of the good days—the easy days—to make that groove just a little bit deeper. Our future self will thank us for it.

ON THIS BRIGHT DAY,
I PRACTICE THE HABITS THAT CONTRIBUTE
TO MY BRIGHT IDENTITY.

THE MAINTENANCE DANCE

> I look for what needs to be done.
> After all, that's how the universe designs itself.
> — R. BUCKMINSTER FULLER

Most of us start Bright Line Eating for the weight loss. And we can fall in love with that phase, failing to recognize that it is only temporary. While we may come for the vanity, hopefully, we ultimately stay for the sanity.

If we really follow the plan, we will find that we have our Bright Transformation and arrive at a place where we are doing the Maintenance dance. This requires us to let go of the fixation on food and weight as a major focus in our lives. It requires us to open our minds and hearts to where else we are going to find meaning, purpose, validation, and service in our lives beyond our food and our weight.

In the realm of food sobriety, the weight-loss phase should be one and done and Maintenance will be your new normal. Initially, learning to inhabit that world can feel uncomfortable and unfamiliar and require just as much support as losing weight did. But in time this new life with its brilliant, broad horizons will feel like home.

ON THIS BRIGHT DAY,

I LEARN TO LET GO OF FOOD AS MY FOCUS
AND LIVE IN PEACE.

LABELS

Everybody is all right really.
— WINNIE-THE-POOH (A. A. MILNE)

Embracing the identity of an addict in recovery can be liberating and can also provide an affiliation with a group of people who are in the same boat. It can help to explain all manner of personality traits, thinking patterns, follies, and foibles that otherwise do not have a good explanation. And it can provide a compelling rationale for working an intensive program of recovery. So for some people it is helpful, comforting, and effective to identify with the label.

Others do not like to think of themselves as food addicts, and that is okay. It does not matter what you call yourself. What matters is that you are honest about the way you eat, the peace of mind you feel, and whether or not your program is working. If you are breaking your Bright Lines regularly, you are probably not working a strong enough program to heal your brain and perhaps are not nourishing yourself in other ways as well. Recognizing what you need to be healthy and well is way more important than using or not using a label. The point is that you work a program that is potent enough to address the challenges and behaviors that you are manifesting.

ON THIS BRIGHT DAY,

I EMBRACE WORKING A PROGRAM THAT IS
STRONG ENOUGH TO SET ME FREE.

December

December 1
PEOPLE PLEASING

---

*To approval addicts, criticism is always highly personal . . .
because people-pleasers . . . cannot clearly distinguish
who they are from what they do.*
— HARRIET BRAIKER

So many of us were unconsciously raised to please those around us. Indeed, our society richly rewards people who are agreeable, helpful, and responsive. And perhaps in our childhood, meeting others' needs first was essential to feeling safe. But seeking approval in adulthood often leads us to ignore what we want and need. It can be hard to stay Bright because that pleasing part of us does not know how to balance the need to belong with the self-care we require.

People-pleasing can keep us from staying Bright in two ways. First, when we are so overcommitted to doing things for others, we do not have time to build food prep, meditation, and social support into our life. Second, we cave when offered NMF. Saying a simple "no, thank you," when people offer us food they have made especially for us requires practice. We do not put anything in our mouths to make someone else happy. That is an old pattern that needs to stop today. The clearer we are about that, the less others will hound us to change our minds.

When we please ourselves by staying Bright, we become someone who has the power to take care of ourselves and others—healthily.

ON THIS BRIGHT DAY,

I WILL TUNE IN TO MYSELF BEFORE AGREEING
TO DO SOMETHING FOR SOMEONE ELSE.

MONITOR YOUR HABITS

---

*If one remains as careful at the end as at the
beginning, there will be no failure.*

— LAO TZU

In the past, we were striving to be the people we wanted to be. We wanted to have a clean and tidy house. We wanted to exercise. We wanted to eat well. We wanted to put ourselves out into the world romantically and professionally with confidence. But our relationship with food made our lives unmanageable. Now we have an opportunity to be the people we always wanted to be. Measuring and monitoring our habits is one of the tools that will help get us there. As we say, *what gets measured gets managed.*

When we track what we are doing in a Nightly Checklist, we have the opportunity to see in reality how we are faring in the program and make improvements—as well as take stock of our accomplishments and consistency. Progress is deeply rewarding, as is the integrity of showing up faithfully. And tallying those daily accomplishments releases dopamine in healthy doses, not addictive doses, which helps keep our brain happy as we progress in this new life. By keeping an eye on ourselves, we build trust, and trust leads to freedom.

ON THIS BRIGHT DAY,

I TRACK AND MONITOR THE HABITS
THAT SERVE ME BEST.

December 3
JFTFP

---

*Make your ego porous. Will is of little importance,
complaining is nothing, fame is nothing. Openness,
patience, receptivity, solitude is everything.*

— RAINER MARIA RILKE

Surrender to the program can sometimes feel elusive. If we are having a hard time manufacturing the feeling of surrender, an effective substitute is to JFTFP—Just Follow the F'ing Plan. JFTFP is something we can choose to do on any given day, and we only ever have to do it *for* today.

Those who follow the plan as is—without substitutions, exceptions, cutting corners, or tinkering—succeed in BLE at a higher rate than those who do not. There is a level of surrender that comes from following what has worked for thousands to successfully lose weight and maintain a healthy body weight from then on.

If you find yourself wanting to make exceptions, get curious about what your motivation is. Are you trying to mimic a food that is not on the BLE plan? Are you trying to speed up weight loss because you are still stuck in a diet mentality? Be curious, and just for today, try following the f'ing plan.

ON THIS BRIGHT DAY,
I WILL RELEASE RESISTANCE AND
FOLLOW THE BLE PLAN.

December 4
WHAT IS THIN?

Satisfaction lies in the effort, not in the attainment,
full effort is full victory.
— MAHATMA GANDHI

When Bright Line Eating first started, "Happy, Thin, and Free" was the tagline, but what we learned is that *thin* is very open to interpretation. Based on where we live in the world and our cultural heritage and even what century we were born in, notions of an ideal body size and shape vary tremendously. The reality is that at some point on our journey, we will need to truly surrender the never-ending striving to be thinner.

Body dissatisfaction is like a pair of glasses that we are going to need to take off to ever have peace. The goal is not objective beauty or even the body that is the best that we can have. The goal is contentment. People who are content in their bodies are attractive and desirable *because* of the peace and confidence they have. Our goal in recovery, above everything, is always that sense of peace, contentment, and confidence in our own skin. *That* is the Bright Transformation.

ON THIS BRIGHT DAY,

I LET GO OF PREVIOUS IDEALS AND PRACTICE
BEING AMAZED AT ALL MY BODY CAN DO.

December 5
CIRCLE OF SUPPORT

Because you know what happens when you say
"hello" or "good morning"? You make a connection.
And isn't that what being human is all about?
— PHILIP ROSENTHAL

Most of us need more support than we think we do. Creating a circle of people in recovery who fully know us and who share this journey with us can buoy up our program immeasurably. Because most people eat for reasons other than hunger, talking about those reasons and life circumstances with others helps us process them, so they don't metastasize and set off cravings. For extroverts, we recommend a circle of at least a dozen people; for introverts, half that works well.

At first the conversations could seem awkward and just be routine. But intimacy develops over time, and through repeated contact we experience how human connection replenishes willpower—and why for so many people on this journey, the best part of the Bright Life is the people we get to travel with.

ON THIS BRIGHT DAY,
I WILL TEND MY GARDEN OF SUPPORT.

December 6
FOCUS ON PEOPLE

People may hear your words, but they feel your attitude.
— JOHN C. MAXWELL

Food obsession is a self-focused, self-centered state of mind, so when we get out of ourselves and think of others, it breaks the stranglehold that food has on us. Now that we are in recovery, we are free to meet others, share ourselves, and be a kind and safe container for those who may not yet be as comfortable as we are.

Focusing on people is an incredibly powerful tool and brings us closer to the true spirit of any holiday. If you find yourself at an event and don't quite know what to do because you are not drinking NMD or eating NMF, look for someone standing alone and ask how they are. Rather than telling a story that entertains or impresses, try being interested in others and watch how we become more interesting ourselves.

A fun challenge is to deliberately meet five people and try to remember their names and three things about each one of them. By making a game of it, this strategy can carry you through a whole event with purpose and amusement. If it is an event where you know people, try asking, "What is new in your world?" and "What has got your attention in life these days?" When we engage with others and ignore the NMF, we leave every encounter enriched—instead of stuffed.

ON THIS BRIGHT DAY,

I WILL FOCUS ON OTHERS AND WATCH MY WORLD BLOSSOM.

December 7
APPRECIATION

Always remember that you are absolutely unique.
Just like everyone else.
— MARGARET MEAD

Harvard professor and Happiness Studies Academy founder Tal Ben-Shahar said, "When you appreciate the good, the good appreciates." Meaning that when we focus on the good in our life, it grows larger with our incredibly powerful magnifying minds.

If we start focusing on the good, it will get bigger and bigger. Appreciation is a muscle that gets stronger with use, an attitude that changes what we see, and an orientation in the world that makes others around us blossom. Be patient with yourself. It takes practice to find the silver lining in an obstacle and something to appreciate about everyone and every situation. And do not forget yourself. Do not wait until you are in your goal body to appreciate your courage, stamina, persistence, and optimism! Appreciate yourself and others and watch what you have to appreciate grow!

ON THIS BRIGHT DAY,
I FOCUS ON WHAT IS UNIQUE AND POSITIVE,
IN OTHERS AND IN MYSELF.

THE NATURAL WORLD

Nature does not hurry.
Yet everything is accomplished.
— LAO TZU

The natural world awaits our interaction and offers itself to us when we enter with curiosity and presence. When we free up space in our life by not focusing on food and dieting anymore, we have more room to form a deeper bond with nature.

Entering a space that fills our heart, either one we have visited or one that lives only in our imagination, can be a perfect pause and centering exercise when a food thought comes up. Studies have shown that just looking at pictures of nature lowers our heartrate and drops our cortisol levels, enabling us to return to our Authentic Self.[9] And when we do our deepest healing work with our wounded inner parts, imagining bringing them to an especially precious place in nature can be a nurturing step in the process of helping them feel safe and whole again.

Fond memories are created in natural settings, so the next time you find yourself somewhere beautiful, take a deep breath, notice all your senses, and savor it. Make a cellular memory to draw upon later in moments of stress.

ON THIS BRIGHT DAY,

I WILL REMEMBER TO DRAW ON THE NOURISHMENT
OF THE NATURAL WORLD.

MODES OF CONNECTION

You cannot truly listen to anyone and
do anything else at the same time.
— M. SCOTT PECK

Because connection is so critical in recovery, we take advantage of every form of connection available to us. As new apps are invented, we find novel ways to link with Bright Lifers all over the world through videos, chats, and text messages. Those who prefer face-to-face encounters start a BLE "Brightest" group in their area or even fly to meet up with their phone buddies in person.

Ultimately, the mode of connection is less important than the quality of the conversation, and BLE worldwide is known for genuine, loving interactions. There are no strangers in BLE. So today explore if there is a new mode of connection you might want to try. If posting online feels too public, maybe start a Slack channel with some BLE friends. If one more app feels overwhelming, start a text thread with your Mastermind Group. If you do not like text threads, try posting online or making a phone call. There are endless options, but all will take you to the same place of loving connection and support.

ON THIS BRIGHT DAY,
I LISTEN WITH ALL MY BEING NO MATTER
WHICH MEDIUM I USE.

December 10

TRUE NOURISHMENT

The name we give to something shapes our attitude toward it.

— KATHERINE PATERSON

Learning to discern what we really want and need is a lifelong process and it is catapulted up a level when we put down sugar and flour and bound our meals and portions. Now we have the space to notice when we have an urge to eat outside of meals and remember that it is not hunger but some other need that has come to the surface. Only when we can notice and name that real need do we have a shot at actually meeting it with true nourishment.

Most needs are met through greater connection—with ourselves, others, a power greater than ourselves, or the natural world. Learning to ask, *What am I really needing here?* and then listening for the best way to meet that need is an exciting adventure. Today ask yourself, *What kind of true nourishment am I seeking in my heart and soul?*

ON THIS BRIGHT DAY,

I WILL NAME MY NEEDS, WANTS, AND DESIRES
AND NOURISH THEM WHOLEHEARTEDLY.

DOING BETTER THAN WE ARE FEELING

When I wake up in a bad mood,
I try not to stay in one. Learn to make
the best of what you have.

— FAITH HILL

The reality of being human is that some days we are just going to feel off, perhaps really off, and we might not know why. Especially when we are in the weight-loss phase.

We truly are detoxing our bodies and healing our brains, and there may be days where that process affects our mood. But if we scan our environment and are left wondering why we are not feeling good, it is critical to take an inventory of our actions. Are we Bright? Is our food in order? How are our habits? Are we staying connected with other people? If we find that we are doing all the right things on our Bright Journey, taking all the actions that support us, then we can take comfort and feel relief. Our moods will catch up because we are doing the right things.

Feelings follow actions. If we are *not* doing the right things, then the good news is that we can take some quick actions to correct the situation and rest easy knowing that we are now doing our part. Our emotional system will catch up soon.

ON THIS BRIGHT DAY,

I FOCUS ON MY ACTIONS AND LET
MY EMOTIONS FOLLOW SUIT.

FIND YOUR TEACHERS

We have a hunger of the mind which asks
for knowledge of all around us, and the more
we gain, the more is our desire; the more we see,
the more we are capable of seeing.
— MARIA MITCHELL

No matter how much we know about any given subject, someone is ahead of us. That is great news because it means we always have someone to lead the way. People love to think that when the student is ready, the teacher appears. But what is also true is that when the student is ready, everyone and everything becomes their teacher.

By getting into a beginner's mindset, you will be willing to learn more about BLE, your journey, your own frame of mind, and skills like meditation and journaling. You will also be able to find someone more skilled or experienced who is happy to share their knowledge with you.

ON THIS BRIGHT DAY,

I NOTICE THE TEACHERS ON MY PATH AND APPRECIATE
WHAT THEY HAVE TO OFFER ME.

DARKEST DAYS

*Even a happy life cannot be without
a measure of darkness.*

— CARL JUNG

As we head toward the winter solstice in the Northern Hemisphere, our days are shortening and we may feel like hibernating. When we are deprived of enlivening sunlight, seasonal affective disorder (SAD) can make some of us feel blue. But even those who do not suffer from SAD may have relied on sugar and flour to cheer ourselves up, especially when so much of it is on offer at the holidays. In the past, this might have meant holing up with NMF and comforting ourselves until spring. What we may find now, though, is that as the depressive effect of sugar leaves our system, we do not feel as sad as we once did during the colder months.

As our bodies heal and release excess weight, we may also find that we have ease in the snow that we did not have before. We may even want to try skiing, snowshoeing, sledding, or ice-skating. Or perhaps a walk in the woods. Just as we replenish when we tuck ourselves in for the night, we can learn to appreciate the beauty of a planet that has the same wisdom. What can you nourish over this coming winter that will blossom for you come spring?

ON THIS BRIGHT DAY,

I LOOK AT THE DARKNESS AS A TIME OF
RENEWAL AND RESTORATION.

December 14
WE ARE NOT OUR PAST

The curious paradox is that
when I accept myself just as I am,
then I can change.
— CARL R. ROGERS

Many of us have lived through some truly harrowing experiences. Some were imposed upon us, but others were the result of our addiction. There are people in this community who have done real harm to their bodies—ruptured their stomachs from bingeing or left themselves with irreparable damage to their esophagi. But no matter how challenging, scarring, traumatizing, or even amazing our history has been, we are not beholden to it or shaped exclusively by these experiences.

The gift of recovery from any addiction is recreating ourselves, rebirthing, and restarting every single day. There is choice in every day, so how do you want to show up in this moment? Which version of yourself would you like to inhabit, because truly, it is a matter of deciding and leaning into it. You are not your past.

ON THIS BRIGHT DAY,

I KNOW MY PAST DOES NOT DEFINE ME,
AND I LEAN INTO BRIGHT CHOICES.

December 15
SHARE ALL OF YOURSELF

I'm not telling you a story so much as a shipwreck—
the pieces floating, finally legible.
— OCEAN VUONG

When we come into food recovery, our life story is often fragmented, and we are still triggered by things that remind our brains of past events. But as we heal over time, our story becomes integrated. What we are likely to find is that the most gruesome parts of our past—the parts that caused us the most grief or pain—can end up being our greatest assets as we use our story to help others. Just as it takes one to know one, it takes one to help one.

In Bright Line Eating, we are able to help others who are experiencing food struggles and life circumstances that are similar to the challenges that we have gone through and survived, especially if we have done our inner work and have integrated and found peace, healing, perspective, and reconciliation. In BLE, you are invited to bring your whole self into the program, to share all aspects of your life, and to be vulnerable, which means sharing all of yourself with someone. Take a risk that someone who is in a similar situation may find hope in your story.

ON THIS BRIGHT DAY,

I WILL SHARE MY STORY WITH SOMEONE I TRUST.

TOOLS ONLY WORK WHEN USED

Experience is that marvelous thing that enables you to recognize a mistake when you make it again.

— FRANKLIN P. JONES

People do not stumble in their recovery because they lack information. They know they need to write down their food, pick up the phone, make connections, meditate, and monitor. But tools are only useful when they are actually used. And in the gap *between* knowledge and action, habits can carry us rather than willpower. Which is why what matters in recovery is our actions, not our knowledge, and not even our desire to do those actions. Success is simply taking the action no matter what, until it becomes automatic.

Our day needs to contain a steady flow of actions that support our recovery. Bright Line Eating has a success rate like no other because it is an integrated system of an effective food plan *with* habits and tools that support human connection. It all works together. If you find yourself not using the BLE tools very often or not taking advantage of the full toolbox, start by noticing which one calls to you and pick that one up. Eventually your repertoire will grow.

ON THIS BRIGHT DAY,

I AVOID A PAST MISTAKE BY USING A NEW TOOL.

SPIRITUAL AND EMOTIONAL FITNESS

> Human freedom involves our capacity to pause, to choose the one response toward which we wish to throw our weight.
>
> — ROLLO MAY

Spiritual and emotional fitness is the buffer zone between what happens in the world and how we respond to it. In other words, when hard things happen, are we able to stick to our Bright Lines and be tolerant and loving? If we have a history of responding to stressors by eating, that can hinder our ability to mature and grow into thoughtful, responsive beings who choose ever more skillful responses to the range of things that can come up during a day.

As we put down the food as our go-to coping mechanism, we are launched on an amazing lifelong journey of becoming ever more skillful at how we respond to life. Can we stay in our Authentic Self—calm, clear, compassionate, confident, connected, curious, courageous, and creative—and respond from that place? If you find yourself not responding but reacting in old ways, you may need to build your emotional and spiritual muscles through meditation, inspirational reading, talking to others, and service to the BLE community. Having your willpower replenished through these channels will give you enough time to pause before choosing your response to life's challenges.

ON THIS BRIGHT DAY,

I LET THE SPACE BETWEEN ACTION
AND REACTION EXPAND.

CHOOSE YOUR HARD

I'm not afraid of storms, for I'm learning how to sail my ship.
— LOUISA MAY ALCOTT

It is important to distinguish between hard in the short term and hard in the long term, and between delayed gratification and instant gratification. While eating our way through life is less hard in the moment because we get to immediately stuff down, wash down, and numb out everything that happens by putting something in our mouth, that path is also often marked by increasing health problems, chronic weight struggles, and feelings of desperation, depression, and low self-esteem.

When we enter recovery, life feels harder because we have to face it in the moment without using food as a crutch. But that short-term difficulty leads to the long-term benefits of living in our Bright Body, feeling like we are the best version of ourself, and enjoying the peace of a life that is well ordered and manageable. There will be some challenges no matter which path you take, but with BLE, at least you are on new terrain and the difficulties will lead you to develop new muscles and new neural pathways that will eventually allow you to summit a mountain with a view you have long yearned to see.

ON THIS BRIGHT DAY,

I CHOOSE THE PATH THAT SERVES ME BEST, NO MATTER HOW HARD IT MAY SEEM RIGHT NOW.

December 19
SILENCE

Silence moves through all sound
like water through netting.
— MARTIN LAIRD

When we ate as our primary reaction to life, we filled all the spaces, including the silence. A lot of us ate while watching TV or while listening to the radio or to a podcast. We wouldn't even allow ourselves to hear the noise of our eating. We needed noise upon noise.

Some of the gifts of a Bright Life are the gift of silence, the gift of spaciousness, and the gift of peace. Do you have enough silence in your day? Do you welcome silence? Avoid it? Listen for it? Silence has a texture that permeates everything, so if you are feeling overwhelmed, consider being silent for just five minutes to pay attention to something that requires your wholehearted presence. The space that eating only three meals a day creates can ripple into other areas, where the spaciousness of silence and listening to your own thoughts becomes a balm for busy times.

ON THIS BRIGHT DAY,

I WILL SAVOR SILENCE.

SINE WAVES ARE HUMAN

It is good to have an end to journey towards;
but it is the journey that matters in the end.
— URSULA K. LE GUIN

The natural shape of life has ups and downs, and the wisdom that comes with age is knowing that our experiences are going to cycle. How steep those highs and lows are, however, is significantly within our control. If we are trending down on that sine wave, we can take actions to shore up our program long before we hit the danger and destruction zone. We do that through reinforcing the habits that keep us nourished and our willpower replenished—the habits of self-care, connection, and service.

We may also recognize that when we are sliding down the slope, it is not the time to expect excellence and a fully checked-off to-do list; rather it's important to put on bunny slippers and have more grace for ourselves. Building in some restorative time is always wise when we feel that things are harder than usual and we are starting to lapse. If you would like a gentler rhythm to your life and would prefer to learn through joy and experience rather than pain and drama, then build in the buffer zone that allows your own sine wave to be just a bit softer.

ON THIS BRIGHT DAY,

I WILL NOTICE IF I AM SLIDING AND TAKE CORRECTIVE
ACTIONS TO MAKE THE JOURNEY GENTLER.

December 21
ENGAGE WITH LIFE

We are not here to amass hoards.
The ants can do that. Rather, we are here to take
those stockpiles and release them into the
energy of generosity and compassion.

— CYNTHIA BOURGEAULT

There is a saying in AA: your addiction just wants you alone—
and then it wants you dead. Using food as an emotional buffer is a self-absorbed and often isolating activity. One of the gifts of living Bright is that we now get to engage fully with others. As this calendar year comes to an end, there are extra opportunities to take advantage of. There are also more stressors, which mean more chances to be there for others in their moment of tension, stress, and need. The more we can keep ourselves Bright, the more we can offer a soft landing place for others when they are going through hardship.

Be the first one to say hi to the stranger, volunteer to help when asked, step forward to be part of the new circle. Fill the hole that sugar or flour once did with kindness and generosity toward others and watch your own life light up.

ON THIS BRIGHT DAY,
I WILL EXTEND MY GENEROSITY TO EVERYONE
WHO CROSSES MY PATH.

December 22
ENLARGE YOUR LIFE

The power that makes grass grow, fruit ripen,
and guides the bird in flight is in us all.
— ANZIA YEZIERSKA

Most of us find our range of focus narrows when we are actively pursuing the next bite of addictive food. BLE helps us broaden our awareness because we no longer have to focus on food. Our daily pattern of Bright living puts food into its proper perspective through giving us few food decisions throughout the day because we have committed our food the night before and know exactly what and when we are going to eat.

Have you put a ceiling on your dreams? Or have you not even allowed yourself to imagine a life that makes your heart sing? This is the time to say yes to the invitations coming to you and the opportunities to use your talents and gifts, as well as to walk the path with new friends you did not even have a year ago.

We do not enlarge our lives overnight, but instead we gradually stretch into them, like they're a new outfit that fits perfectly but is in a new style we never imagined would look so good on us.

ON THIS BRIGHT DAY,

I TAP INTO THE POWER WITHIN MYSELF TO MOVE
IN THE DIRECTION OF MY CHOOSING.

BREATHE, PRAY, CALL

At the innermost core of all loneliness is a deep
and powerful yearning for union with one's lost self.
— BRENDAN FRANCIS BEHAN

An Emergency Action Plan is something we have ready for when life gets lifey and we want to eat off plan. A simple plan like *breathe, pray, call* can be memorized and become a mantra of guidance when we are rattled. First, we breathe deeply, bringing our awareness into our body, a grounding action that returns us into the present moment and the only place from which we can make an authentic decision. Second, we pray. Praying works for those who have a belief in something greater than themselves, but it also works for those who do not because articulating the need out loud or clearly within the mind to the Authentic Self can be hugely helpful. Third, we call someone so we are not debating our inner Indulger by ourselves, a fight that we will typically lose alone. We enlist a calm, wise other who can help remind us why it is so much better to stick to the Bright Lines.

The next time you find yourself getting seduced by NMF, breathe, pray, and call—and watch yourself emerge Brighter and available for the next chance encounter.

ON THIS BRIGHT DAY,

I WILL PAUSE WHEN I AM OFF CENTER,
AND BREATHE, PRAY, AND CALL.

December 24
SEASONS

The only thing that's really worthwhile is change. It's coming.
— SEPTIMA POINSETTE CLARK

All endeavors have seasons. Perhaps our recovery journey came easily to us in the summer when our local farm stand made shopping for vegetables fun. Maybe we enjoyed meeting up with fellow Bright Lifers and going for outdoor walks. For some, the winter can feel isolating as the ground hardens and the days shorten. For others, the winter offers an opportunity to strengthen their program without the social distractions of summer.

For every person, there are seasons of connection, solitude, socializing, and reflection. Honoring them all, listening to your inner guidance, and being curious about your motivation for any action or inaction will help put the fluctuations of life in perspective. No matter how you feel about this season, remember that a season is only a period of time that will pass and that it has its own unique gifts to offer us.

What can you celebrate about hibernation? What can this season offer you?

ON THIS BRIGHT DAY,

I HONOR THE SEASONS IN NATURE, IN MY BODY,
AND IN MY LIFE.

December 25

JOY

Focus on the journey, not the destination.
Joy is found not in finishing an activity but in doing it.
— GREG ANDERSON

Joy does not depend on an external context but rather is a deep state of being, an orientation toward the world and self that is based on believing that all is well, people are fundamentally good, and life has meaning. Looking for that meaning, being of service, and leaning into connections all create joy for us.

We each have a set point for joy. If we want to raise it, gratitude is an invaluable practice. When we look at all the things that are well in our world, we can feel an enormous surge. Being attentive to small moments of joy can also increase our capacity. We can create a moment of joy with another person through sharing the briefest glance or a warm smile.

If today is hard, if you are far from family, if today is not a holiday for you, or if you are struggling through your first Christmas without NMF, notice those who seem more consistently joyful and learn what they do and think. Tune into gratitude. And lean into community.

ON THIS BRIGHT DAY,

I CELEBRATE THE JOY THAT I DERIVE
FROM MY CONNECTIONS, MY CLARITY,
AND MY SELF-COMPASSION.

A BIG ENOUGH CONVERSATION

It always comes back to the same necessity:
go deep enough and there is a bedrock of truth,
however hard.

— MAY SARTON

Are you talking about big ideas, the things you really believe, and sharing stories that matter? It is so easy to get bogged down in the logistics and transactional conversations of daily life, especially with those who live in our household. Setting aside time for more contemplative, humorous, and philosophical conversations can be nourishing and grounding. Even if we only have those conversations with ourselves and our journal, it is vital to think about what has meaning for us and where the depth is in our life.

As the New Year approaches, we want to start thinking about the big questions, to ask ourselves if there are any shifts that we want to make. What are we working on in our growth trajectory right now? So today, skip the small talk and ask someone a Big Question. And answer their Big Question with candor and vulnerability. You may be surprised where the conversation will lead you.

ON THIS BRIGHT DAY,

I WELCOME THE DEEPEST CONNECTIONS AVAILABLE.

December 27
COUNTING DAYS

All great achievements require time.
— MAYA ANGELOU

As we come to the end of the calendar year, we may be taking stock. Was this a Bright year? Was it a Bright month? Week? Some of us count our Bright Days to motivate ourselves and add to our momentum. Many know the exact date we started eating Bright and celebrate anniversaries and milestones. Some people only count days that are completely Bright; if they break their Lines, rather than resetting to zero, they keep counting minus the day of the break. If starting at zero after Rezooming fills you with shame, don't do it. If it fills you with resolve and hope, then by all means.

You do your program the way that works best for your peace of mind and well-being. But if this was a year when you tried to orient toward this way of life, however much you may have struggled, then it was a Brightening year. Your life is Brightening. And next year will be Brighter still. As you reflect, try not to focus on the dark patches of struggle, but rather on the light you brought to your life and the lives of others. Count your commitment and watch it grow.

ON THIS BRIGHT DAY,

I WILL HAVE PRIDE FOR EACH BRIGHT MEAL
BECAUSE IT MATTERS.

KEEP FOOD BLACK AND WHITE

Truth is ever to be found in the simplicity,
not in the multiplicity and confusion of things.

— SIR ISAAC NEWTON

When we were trying to get much of our life satisfaction from food, we were left in an endless cycle of wanting and yearning and craving. Food can only take us so far. One of the benefits of having crisp Bright Lines, a list of foods that are BLE friendly, and a clear program of action, is that we now have so much more energy, space, and actual time to use for other areas of life. The saying "I keep my food black and white, so I can live in color" means having the addiction handled, one day at a time, so that we can lean into the wonder that is available in every human interaction.

The reality is that the color, vibrancy, excitement, satisfaction, contentment, and comfort that we were looking to get from our food is simply not available there. While keeping our food black and white may feel terrifying at first, it is in truth the path to the vibrancy we seek.

ON THIS BRIGHT DAY,

I LEAN INTO THE CLARITY OF MY LINES AND LOOK
FOR EXCITEMENT ELSEWHERE.

December 29
FOCUS ON THE LINES

To live only for some future goal is shallow.
It's the sides of the mountain that sustain life, not the top.
— ROBERT M. PIRSIG

"If you focus on your Bright Lines you will lose the weight; if you focus on the weight you will lose your Bright Lines."

This saying proves useful whenever obsession with our weight threatens to shift us from a recovery mentality to a diet mentality. We need to be in this for the long haul because fundamentally, we are going to keep doing this the same way once we are living in our Bright Body and for years and decades beyond that. If that is not our plan, this is all nothing more than a diet, where we do it for a time and then stop and gain all our weight back eventually.

It does not matter whether it takes us two months or two years to be in whatever we would consider a Bright Body. The blessed reality is that once we have a little bit of Bright time under our belt, we are in a Bright Body anyway. We are in a body that is being nourished with Bright food, living a Bright Life, and focused on Bright pursuits.

ON THIS BRIGHT DAY,
I WILL SETTLE IN FOR THE JOURNEY KNOWING
THAT THIS PATH IS THE WAY I CHOOSE TO TRAVEL.

December 30
INTIMACY

Real intimacy is only possible to the
degree that we can be honest about what
we are doing and feeling.
— JOYCE BROTHERS

As we renegotiate a relationship with ourselves, we may need to relearn what it means to be intimate—with ourselves and others. A critical part of ourselves may have prevented us from even enjoying our own touch or that of others. Now is the time to explore and permeate those old boundaries.

We take time in the shower to stay present and feel all of ourselves. We learn to love our bodies by rubbing lotion on our skin in a way that feels both nourishing and sensual. We slip into fabrics that make us aware of our skin's pleasure receptors. And we allow ourselves the vulnerability of being touched by a partner.

Emotional intimacy means no longer using food to bond with others but rather creating bonds through talking and sharing and listening and laughing, far more profound sources of connection. We find the intimacy within by sitting in meditation and occupying the vast blackness of our mind, breathing into that space in our body deeply for many long, silent minutes. See how you can explore your own brave intimacy today.

ON THIS BRIGHT DAY,
I REVEL IN MOMENTS OF AUTHENTIC INTIMACY
WITH MYSELF AND OTHERS.

December 31
IMPACT

No individual has any right to come into the world
and go out of it without leaving behind distinct and
legitimate reasons for having passed through it.
— GEORGE WASHINGTON CARVER

Whatever we think the meaning of life is, most of us want to have a positive impact on the world, especially on the people around us. Getting Bright has a powerful impact on our sense of self. When we live in alignment with our food, eating only and exactly what we commit to eat, we find that we start to radiate the calm, confident, centered air of someone who makes the best choices for themselves over and over. From that new-found sense of integrity, we then become a beacon of hope for the people in our community. From there we can step out into the world, making an impact through our profession, our vocation, our avocation, the family we are raising, and the way we move through our lives. But it all starts with the daily commitment to this Bright path. From there we are unstoppable.

ON THIS BRIGHT DAY,

I MAKE CHOICES THAT SUPPORT MY RECOVERY
AND WATCH THE RIPPLES SPREAD TO OTHERS.

RESOURCES

To take the quiz to discover how susceptible your brain is to the addictive properties of ultra-processed foods, visit:

https://FoodAddictionQuiz.com

To download the Emergency Action Plan, the Nightly Checklist, and the Permission to Be Human Action Plan, visit:

https://OnThisBrightDay.com

To access a treasure trove of free video support for your journey (the weekly VLOG archives) and learn how to join with a community of like-minded people doing Bright Line Eating and living their Brightest Lives, visit:

https://BrightLineEating.com

To find a 12-step meeting for food addiction or compulsive overeating, or to access audio recordings of people who have found freedom from food obsession, visit:

https://FoodAddicts.org (FA, for food addicts)

https://OA.org (OA, for compulsive overeaters)

GLOSSARY

Authentic Self—in Internal Family Systems Therapy, the person we are when we are our true selves. We know we are operating from this seat of highest self when we feel calm, clear, compassionate, confident, creative, curious, courageous, and connected.

BLE—(see Bright Line Eating)

BLTs (Bites, Licks, and Tastes)—food snuck during meal preparation or eaten off others' plates

Bright Bodies—come in a range of shapes and sizes. Their underlying commonality is that they are free of processed sugar and flour, have shed their unhealthy weight, and carry minds that are at peace with food and focused outward on the world at large.

Bright Community—the online and in-person global network of people doing Bright Line Eating

Bright Lifer—a member of the Bright community whose sense of identity is inextricably linked with following the four Bright Lines in BLE

Bright Line—a clear, unambiguous boundary that you never cross. Example: a nonsmoker never smokes cigarettes.

Bright Line Eating (BLE)—a method of eating where four Bright Lines are rigorously followed: no sugar, no flour, no excess quantities, and no eating between meals

Bright Transformation—the weight loss and complete physical, mental, emotional, and spiritual change that accompanies adhering to the four Bright Lines and working the BLE program

Buddy—a person in the BLE community with whom a Bright Lifer shares a bilateral dynamic of support

Committing—the act of sharing precisely what will be eaten for the day with the online support community, a Guide, a Buddy, a supportive human being, or God

Emergency Action Plan (EAP)—the series of steps a Bright Lifer plans to take when food cravings hit. Common steps include taking three deep breaths, praying for the cravings to be removed, writing a gratitude list, going for a walk, and calling a Buddy. Bright Lifers often write their EAP down and carry it with them.

Food Addiction Susceptibility Quiz—(see Susceptibility Quiz)

Food Addiction Susceptibility Scale—(see Susceptibility Scale)

Guide—another Bright Lifer who helps us through a short-term phase or challenge such as Rezooming or transitioning to Maintenance

Internal Family Systems (IFS) Therapy—operates from the premise that the psyche has parts, which can be in harmony or in conflict. These parts typically came into being as coping mechanisms in childhood, and they do the best they can with the tools they have.

> **Inner Caretaker**—serves others at the expense of caring for ourselves
>
> **Inner Controller**—thrives on micromanaging our food and weight
>
> **Inner Indulger**—wants to soothe and reward us with NMF and NMD
>
> **Inner Isolator**—pulls us away from getting the support we need
>
> **Inner Rebel**—bucks against restrictions

Maintenance—once Bright Lifers have shed their excess weight, they transition to this stage where they eat the exact amount of food required to maintain their weight in their goal range and make them feel energetic and peaceful. Food is often added to or subtracted from a Maintenance Food Plan as weight drifts down or up. This stage lasts a lifetime.

Mastermind Group—a small group who meets regularly to support one another's Bright Journeys

Nightly Checklist—a tracking tool, whether digital or analog, for recording daily adherence to Bright Lines and support tools

NMD (Not My Drink)—any beverage outside a person's Bright Line Eating plan, most typically one containing alcohol. NMD can also refer to beverages containing sugar, artificial sweeteners, caffeine, or calories.

NMF (Not My Food)—junk food or food containing sugar and/or flour. A food can be sugar- and flour-free but still classified as NMF if it is outside of mealtime or in excess quantities.

Permission-to-Be-Human Action Plan—a list of 10 questions for journaling and reflection after a break in the Bright Lines

Rezoom—after a break (or bend) in one of the Bright Lines, to resume eating Bright as quickly as possible, with the next meal or even the next bite, hence re-*zoom!*

Susceptibility Scale—a scale from 1–10 that measures how strongly people experience food cravings, loss of control over how much they eat, and repeated failures to manage their eating. People who score 9 and 10 on the scale tend to test positive for food addiction; people who score 7 or 8 may as well.

Susceptibility Quiz—available at FoodAddictionQuiz.com, this tool helps people learn where they fall on the Susceptibility Scale, meaning how susceptible they are to the pull of addictive foods

ENDNOTES

1. P. J. Kenny and P. M. Johnson, "Dopamine D2 Receptors in Addiction-like Reward Dysfunction and Compulsive Eating in Obese Rats," *Nature Neuroscience* 13, no. 5 (May 2010): 635–641, doi:10.1038/nn.2519.

2. Y. Ikemi and S. Nakagawa, "A Psychosomatic Study of Contagious Dermatitis," *Kyushu Journal of Medical Science* 13 (1962): 335–350.

3. H. B. Kappes and G. Oettingen, "Positive Fantasies about Idealized Futures Sap Energy," *Journal of Experimental Social Psychology* 47, no. 4 (2011): 719–729.

4. Richard Wiseman, "The Luck Factor," *The Skeptical Inquirer*, May/June 2003, http://www.richardwiseman.com/resources/The_Luck_Factor.pdf.

5. International Diabetes Federation. (2015). IDF DIABETES ATLAS, (7th ed., p. 79). Retrieved from http://www.indiaenvironmentportal.org.in/files/file/IDF_Atlas%202015_UK.pdf.

6. Haijang Dai, et al., "Global, Regional, and National Burden of Ischaemic Heart Disease and Its Attributable Risk Factors, 1990–2017: Results from the Global Burden of Disease Study 2017," *European Heart Journal Quality of Care and Clinical Outcomes* 8, no. 1 (October 5, 2020): 50–60, doi:10.1093/ehjqcco/qcaa076.

7. Eva Ose Askvik, F. R. van der Weel, and Audrey van der Meer, "The Importance of Cursive Handwriting over Typewriting for Learning in the Classroom: A High-Density EEG Study of 12-Year-Old Children and Young Adults," *Journal of Educational Psychology* 11 (July 2020), https://doi.org/10.3389/fpsyg.2020.01810.

8. Deborah W. Tang, Lesley K. Fellows, and Alain Dagher, "Behavioral and Neural Valuation of Foods Is Driven by Implicit Knowledge of Caloric Content," *Psychological Science* 25, no. 12 (October 2014), https://doi.org/10.1177/0956797614552081.

9. Magdalena van den Berg, et al., "Autonomic Nervous System Responses to Viewing Green and Built Settings: Differentiating Between Sympathetic and Parasympathetic Activity," *International Journal of Environmental Research and Public Health* 12, no. 12 (December 2015): 15860–74, doi: 10.3390/ijerph121215026.

ACKNOWLEDGMENTS

This book was the seed of an idea several years ago when I was far too busy to think of hundreds of topics, much less find quotes and write blurbs. But the incomparable JoAnn Campbell-Rice, one of our esteemed Bright Line Eating coaches, joyfully tackled the project. A short time later she delivered a massive collection of ideas. It was an extraordinary feat. As I commenced to write this book some two years later, what I found was that the breadth of vision and the quality of thought JoAnn poured into that compilation made my job ridiculously easy. And, surprisingly, fun. JoAnn, thank you. Oh my goodness, *thank you*. My deepest bow to you.

With book number four, some automaticity has developed. Or at least less insanity. If (for some reason) you've carefully read the acknowledgments in each of my previous books, you will certainly find familiar names and themes. I stay with my adored publishing team because they are maestros of execution, and the love and respect keep deepening. And so, with endless gratitude and appreciation, I once again am privileged to thank . . .

My beloved Nicola of The Finished Thought. You. Are. The. Best. Anyone who is trying to write a book without you in their corner is just kidding themselves. And spinning their wheels. And surely being far too wordy. You carried me through this project with ease and joy and right-on-point deadlines. God, I love you.

My incomparable agent, Lucinda Halpern. Experience, meet class, grace, and brains. We're cruising along together now, arm-in-arm, truly unstoppaBLE. It is my hope that anyone who is trying to negotiate a book deal has your wise counsel over tea. I'm so lucky!

Ashley Bernardi . . . ooooooooh!!! Nowhere was PR more squeal-a-licious than with Nardi Media! You get it done, girlfriend! Podcasts, radio, TV, and print, oh my! Let's keep working together forever, can we?

The Hay House team, starting with Patty Gift and Reid Tracy. I so love being a Hay House author! Thank you for seeking me out and inviting me to join the family. I am blessed. Lisa Cheng, you made this book better; we had to compromise, and we found the sweet spot. Monica O'Connor, Lisa Vega, Julie Davison, Kirsten Callais, Tricia Breidenthal, Celeste Johnson, Lisa Bernier, Steve Morris, Lizzi Marshall, and Lindsay McGinty, thank you for your support, your excellence, and for chasing me down so we could stay on track.

Angela Denby, there is no one whose eye I trust more. You set the bar—the best graphic designer anywhere and so unbelievably wonderful to work with. When people say "talent," they mean you.

Jenn Moon, our proofreader extraordinaire, your eagle eye is unparalleled. Thank you for helping in the most critical week. Because of your talent and skill, I trusted I didn't have to read it yet again. I knew you were on it.

Lori Lang, my partner in crafting the launch of this precious little book into the world. A full year ago you were eagerly stockpiling book launch ideas. And we did it!!! You are so great to work with. I don't know a more kind and lovely soul.

The Bright Line Eating Team. You rock!!! You collaborate, execute, fill gaps, follow through, and love life, each other, and the people we serve all along the way. The smartest, most heart-centered group of professionals anywhere. I pinch myself.

All the brave, amazing people who walk this path of structured eating and Bright living. My beloved Bright Line Eaters, Bright Lifers, and all the members of the many 12-Step food programs, I honor your willingness to let go of toxic, ultra-processed foods and find a new and better way to live. Serving you is my honor. You make me want to rise and find yet more ways to help, educate the masses, and get the word out so that those who are willing to do what it takes won't have to suffer anymore.

My inner circle of support, because holy smokadoodles, I need a lot of support. Christine Gimeno-Davis, Linden Morris Delrio, Cathy Cox, Diana Brewer, Georgia Whitney, Sage Lavine, Ocean Robbins, Everett Considine, Daniel Maggio, Tosca Lindberg, Dana Oliver, Kennedy Wilson, Diane Raike, Shira Coleman Hagar, and Shiraz Nerenberg. My life works because you pick up the phone.

And finally, my favorite people. David—my partner, my ballast, my soul's warm home; Mom and Dad—I explode with love for you; and my precious Zoe, Robin, and Maya—my greatest hopes and best teachers. I could do nothing without your encouragement, support, and sacrifices. You make life rich and full. I love you.

ABOUT THE AUTHOR

SUSAN **P**EIRCE **T**HOMPSON, **P**H.**D**., is the *New York Times* best-selling author of *Bright Line Eating, The Official Bright Line Eating Cookbook*, and *Rezoom*. She is an Adjunct Associate Professor of Brain and Cognitive Sciences at the University of Rochester and an expert in the psychology of eating. She is president of the Institute for Sustainable Weight Loss and the founder of Bright Line Eating, a worldwide movement on a mission to help one million people have their Bright Transformations—the full physical, mental, spiritual, and emotional transformation that accompanies healthy, sustainable weight loss—by 2030. She lives in Rochester, New York, with her husband and their three kiddos.

You can visit her online at SusanPeirceThompson.com or BrightLineEating.com

INDEX

Note: Terms and phrases in *italics* indicate meditations.

Hay House Titles of Related Interest

We hope you enjoyed this Hay House book. If you'd like to receive our online catalog featuring additional information on Hay House books and products, or if you'd like to find out more about the Hay Foundation, please contact:

Hay House, Inc., P.O. Box 5100, Carlsbad, CA 92018-5100
(760) 431-7695 or (800) 654-5126
(760) 431-6948 (fax) or (800) 650-5115 (fax)
www.hayhouse.com® • www.hayfoundation.org

———

Published in Australia by: Hay House Australia Pty. Ltd.,
18/36 Ralph St., Alexandria NSW 2015
Phone: 612-9669-4299 • *Fax:* 612-9669-4144
www.hayhouse.com.au

Published in the United Kingdom by: Hay House UK, Ltd.,
The Sixth Floor, Watson House, 54 Baker Street, London W1U 7BU
Phone: +44 (0)20 3927 7290 • *Fax:* +44 (0)20 3927 7291
www.hayhouse.co.uk

Published in India by: Hay House Publishers India,
Muskaan Complex, Plot No. 3, B-2, Vasant Kunj, New Delhi 110 070
Phone: 91-11-4176-1620 • *Fax:* 91-11-4176-1630
www.hayhouse.co.in

———

Access New Knowledge.
Anytime. Anywhere.

Learn and evolve at your own pace
with the world's leading experts.

www.hayhouseU.com

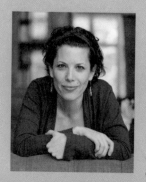

Susan Peirce Thompson, Ph.D., is the *New York Times* best-selling author of *Bright Line Eating, The Official Bright Line Eating Cookbook*, and *Rezoom*. She is an Adjunct Associate Professor of Brain and Cognitive Sciences at the University of Rochester and an expert in the psychology of eating. She is president of the Institute for Sustainable Weight Loss and the founder of Bright Line Eating, a worldwide movement on a mission to help one million people have their Bright Transformations—the full physical, mental, spiritual, and emotional transformation that accompanies healthy, sustainable weight loss—by 2030. She lives in Rochester, New York, with her husband and their three kiddos. You can visit her online at SusanPeirceThompson.com or BrightLineEating.com.

Hay House USA
P.O. Box 5100, Carlsbad, CA 92018-5100
(760) 431-7695 or (800) 654-5126
(760) 431-6948 (fax) or (800) 650-5115 (fax)
www.hayhouse.com®

Front-cover design: Julie Davison
Case design: Lisa Vega
Photo of author: Mike Martinez / Fish & Crown Creative

Printed in the United States of America